SEX
EDUCATION

Other Books in the At Issue Series:

SEX EDUCATION

Tamara L. Roleff, *Book Editor*

David Bender, *Publisher*
Bruno Leone, *Executive Editor*

Bonnie Szumski, *Editorial Director*
Brenda Stalcup, *Managing Editor*
Scott Barbour, *Senior Editor*

613.9
c.2

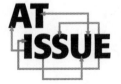

An Opposing Viewpoints® Series

Greenhaven Press, Inc.
San Diego, California

No part of this book may be reproduced or used in any form or by any means, electrical, mechanical, or otherwise, including, but not limited to, photocopy, recording, or any information storage and retrieval system, without prior written permission from the publisher.

Library of Congress Cataloging-in-Publication Data

Sex education / Tamara L. Roleff, book editor.
    p.   cm. — (At issue) (An opposing viewpoints series)
    Reprinted articles.
    Includes bibliographical references and index.
    ISBN 0-7377-0008-4 (pbk. : alk. paper). —
ISBN 0-7377-0009-2 (lib. : alk. paper)
    1. Sex instruction. I. Roleff, Tamara L., 1959– . II. Series: At issue (San Diego, Calif.) III. Series: Opposing viewpoints series (Unnumbered)
HQ56.S376   1999
613.9'071—dc21   98-35008
                                                                                            CIP

©1999 by Greenhaven Press, Inc., PO Box 289009,
San Diego, CA 92198-9009

Printed in the U.S.A.

Every effort has been made to trace owners of copyrighted material.

Table of Contents

Introduction

During the 1960s, the John Birch Society, an ultraconservative organization, pushed schools to eliminate sex education programs in classrooms, charging that the classes were "smut," "immoral," and "a filthy communist plot" to poison the minds of American children. By the end of the 1970s, only the District of Columbia and three states—Kentucky, Maryland, and New Jersey—required that sex education be taught in public schools. The decline in sex education programs in the 1970s was accompanied by a steady increase in the teen sex rate and out-of-wedlock births. When the AIDS epidemic began to expand its reach into America's schools in the 1980s, parents and educators decided that they needed to teach their children about the realities of sex and disease. By December 1997, nineteen states and the District of Columbia required schools to teach sexuality education, and thirty-four states and the District of Columbia required instruction about HIV, AIDS, and other sexually transmitted diseases.

In the mid-1990s, teen sex and illegitimacy became a focus of concern for conservatives who were trying to reform the welfare system. They charged that the welfare system rewarded premarital sex and out-of-wedlock births by granting benefits to unwed mothers. The best way to reduce the welfare rolls, and therefore illegitimacy, they argued, was to emphasize abstinence-only sex education programs in schools. In 1996, Congress included in its welfare reform act a provision to encourage states to require abstinence-only sex education programs in their schools. Congress authorized grants of $250 million over five years to states that required school-based abstinence-only sex education programs. In addition, the five states that showed the largest drop in teen pregnancy without a corresponding increase in the abortion rate would split an additional $400 million.

The 1996 legislation is very specific about what the abstinence-only programs must and must not teach. Under the law, states are mandated to teach that "abstinence from sexual activity outside of marriage is the expected standard"; that "abstinence from sexual activity is the only certain way to avoid out-of-wedlock pregnancy, sexually transmitted diseases, and other associated health problems"; that "a mutually faithful monogamous relationship in the context of marriage is the expected standard of human sexual activity"; that "sexual activity outside of the context of marriage is likely to have harmful psychological and physical effects"; and that "bearing children out-of-wedlock is likely to have harmful consequences for the child, the child's parents, and society." Furthermore, the law prohibits the states from using any of the grant money to teach about contraception or about how students can protect themselves from sexually transmitted diseases (STDs).

Supporters argue that abstinence-only sex education programs instill values in their children and teach them how to say "no" to sex. Supporting their argument is a study by sexuality experts that found that 84 percent of young girls surveyed said they wanted to learn "how to say 'no' to sex without hurting the other person's feelings." Advocates of teen-abstinence programs also assert that teaching youth about birth control in effect gives them permission to engage in premarital sex. According to Elayne Bennett, founder of a national abstinence mentoring program, Best Friends:

> Sex is a serious business, and it's for adults only. When one spends a lot of time instructing teens on all the various paraphernalia for protecting themselves, the message is that it's perfectly safe to do this as long as you protect yourself. But we know that [using protection] does not protect against many STDs.

Teenagers receive a mixed message, Bennett maintains, when they are told how to protect themselves from pregnancy and STDs, yet told that they should remain chaste until marriage.

For abstinence supporters, the failure rate of many birth control methods compounds the problematic message of sex education. According to obstetrician Joe S. McIlhaney Jr., founder of the Medical Institute for Sexual Health, not only do condoms have a high failure rate for preventing STDs, but they also have a high failure rate for preventing pregnancy. A study by researcher Susan C. Weller found that condoms failed to prevent pregnancy up to 13 percent of the time and failed to protect against AIDS and other STDs 31 percent of the time. McIlhaney adds that many married couples do not use condoms correctly, so it is unlikely that inexperienced teens could do so, especially when they are under the influence of drugs or alcohol. The only method guaranteed to prevent pregnancy and STDs is abstinence, he asserts. "The best that 'safer sex' approaches can offer is some risk reduction. Abstinence, on the other hand, offers risk elimination," McIlhaney writes.

McIlhaney and his followers contend that abstinence programs are effective at reducing the teen sex and teen pregnancy rates. For example, they point to a Chicago middle school in which each class had several girls who were pregnant every year. But after three years of an abstinence program, the school graduated three classes in a row in which no girls were pregnant. In Washington, D.C., only 5 percent of the girls in the Best Friends program had ever had sexual intercourse, compared to 63 percent citywide. The Centers for Disease Control and Prevention (CDC) confirmed in June 1998 that the national teen pregnancy rate has been falling since 1990. The center reported that the teen pregnancy rate between 1990 and 1995 dropped from 55 percent to 50 percent without a corresponding increase in the abortion rate. Supporters cite this trend in the falling teen birth rate to support their argument that abstinence-only education is effective.

Supporters of comprehensive sex education programs, in which students are taught about birth control methods and how to protect themselves against STDs, contend that abstinence-only programs are ineffective. Most schools with abstinence-only programs had not implemented the curriculum by 1995, they assert, so the programs cannot take credit for reducing the teen pregnancy rate. Furthermore, according to some sex educators, statistics show that more teens, not fewer, are having sex. The pregnancy rate has declined because more teens are using birth control, they maintain, not because fewer teens are having sex. In fact, birth control proponents point out that the number of teenagers who used condoms during their first sexual experience tripled between 1975 and 1995, from 18 percent to 54 percent.

The CDC contends that birth control methods are much more reliable than their critics claim. Condoms are "highly effective" against AIDS when used correctly and consistently, the center asserts, and fail less than 2 percent of the time. Henry Foster, Bill Clinton's advisor on teen pregnancy, maintains that teens who are not taught the facts about contraception "don't have the facts on how to protect themselves, yet they are bombarded with media messages" that urge them to "just do it." In addition, many sex educators believe that the anti-contraception message may give youth the impression that all forms of safe sex are ineffective, thus leading teens to stop using condoms and other forms of birth control altogether. Such a move would lead to higher pregnancy and STD rates, sex educators claim.

Comprehensive sex education advocates also dispute claims that abstinence-only programs are effective at reducing teen sex and pregnancy rates. Douglas Kirby, a sex education researcher who studied thirty-three sex education programs, found that all six of the abstinence-only programs in his study failed to delay sexual activity. The best documented abstinence-only sex education program was used by California schools from 1992 to 1995. The state spent $15 million over three years teaching abstinence-only to 187,000 middle school students. Kirby found the students who had not participated in abstinence-only classes were no less likely to postpone sexual intercourse or prevent pregnancies or STDs than students who had participated in abstinence-only classes. Kirby's study also found that comprehensive sex education programs do not promote sexual activity. According to Kirby, "Sexuality- and HIV-education curricula do not increase sexual intercourse, either by hastening the onset of intercourse, increasing the frequency of intercourse, or increasing the number of sexual partners."

Most sex educators agree that the most effective programs in reducing teen sex and teen pregnancy combine the information on values from the abstinence curricula and the safe sex information from comprehensive sex education programs. Moreover, polls show that most parents want their children to be taught about contraception. However, this consensus has not stopped the debate over which type of sex education should be taught in public schools. *At Issue: Sex Education* examines the morality and effectiveness of abstinence-only versus comprehensive sex education programs, as well as other sexuality issues.

1

Sex Education Should Be Taught in Schools

Joycelyn Elders interviewed by Priscilla Pardini

Joycelyn Elders is the former surgeon general of the United States. She was forced to resign in December 1994 after commenting that children should be taught about masturbation in schools. Elders is on the staff at Children's Hospital in Little Rock, Arkansas, and on the faculty at the School of Medicine at the University of Arkansas. She is also working on a book, The Dreaded M Word. *Elders was interviewed by Priscilla Pardini, a freelance writer, for* Rethinking Schools, *a periodical that discusses education issues.*

Teens should be taught a comprehensive sex education program that gives them all the facts they need to know about preventing pregnancy and disease. Although parents should ideally be the ones to teach their children about sex, many adults are unable to talk frankly to their children.

What's wrong with abstinence-only sexuality education programs?
Nothing, in the very early grades. If we did a really good job in the first 10 or 12 years of children's lives teaching them about abstinence, as well as about honesty and integrity and responsibility and how to make good decisions, we would not have to be talking to them at 15 about not getting engaged in sex.

But we haven't done that. Mothers have been teaching abstinence, schools have been teaching abstinence, preachers have been preaching abstinence for years. Yet more than three million teens get STDs every year, and we still have the highest teen pregnancy, abortion, and birth rates in the industrialized world. But we seem to feel that we don't need to educate our children about their sexuality. That makes absolutely no sense. We all know the vows of abstinence break far more easily than latex condoms.

Teens need a comprehensive sexuality program that gives them all the information they need to become empowered and responsible for preventing pregnancy and disease. We have to stop trying to legislate morals

Reprinted from Priscilla Pardini, "Vows of Abstinence Break More Easily Than Latex Condoms: An Interview with Joycelyn Elders," *Rethinking Schools*, vol. 12, no. 4 (Summer 1998), by permission of *Rethinking Schools*, 1001 E. Keefe Ave., Milwaukee, WI 53212; 414-964-9646.

and instead teach responsibility. Abstinence-only does not do that. You can't be responsible if you don't have the information.

But is school the best place for sexuality education? Isn't this better left to parents?

I have no problem leaving it to parents, if you have parents who can and will do it. But we have many dysfunctional parents—some on drugs, some into alcohol, some who are stressed out, and some who just don't know how to talk to their children about sex. Then the responsibility belongs to the community. And since the only place we've got access to every child is in school, we need to use our schools to teach about sexuality. We don't depend on parents to teach math and English and science and geography. So why should we depend on parents to teach children all of their social and behavioral skills?

Teachers say they don't have enough time as it is to adequately cover academic subjects. Doesn't sexuality education cut into precious time now allotted to basics such as reading and math?

I think teachers are doing a wonderful job—the best they can under difficult circumstances. But what good is knowing math and science if you don't know how to protect yourself? The fact is, we invest more money in prisons than we do in schools. We're putting out a dragnet when we ought to be putting out a safety net.

Our children, from the time they enter kindergarten through 12th grade, spend 18,000 hours watching TV, but only 12,000 hours in reading and math classes and only 46 hours in health education classes. I say let's take away some of the TV time—and devote more hours to the school day, to summer school.

How early should sexuality education start? What kinds of topics should be covered in the early years?

As early as kindergarten children need to be taught to respect their bodies, to eat in healthy ways and to feel good about themselves. They need to know how to make good decisions and how to deal with conflict in non-violent ways. People who feel good about themselves feel in control of their lives and can make decisions that are right for them. Years later, these children, if they choose to be sexually active, will probably also choose to use a latex condom to protect themselves. But if you're not in control of your sexuality, you can't control your life. Those are the people who end up saying, "It just happened."

We all know vows of abstinence break far more easily than latex condoms.

How can teachers evaluate whether material is age-appropriate for their students? Can you offer some guidelines for elementary, middle and high school?

There are a lot of high-quality, well-tested curricula out there that are age-appropriate. Even very young kids should know that anytime anyone touches you in a way you don't want to be touched, even if it is your parents, you have to tell somebody. That message needs to start in kindergarten, but also needs to be repeated and reinforced. Older kids should learn about the menstrual cycle, that if they choose to be sexually active they can get diseases or get pregnant. They should know that you can get pregnant the first time you have sex . . . that you can get pregnant if you have sex standing up.

By high school, you need to be teaching them more about responsibility and equality—that boys and girls have equal responsibility for their sexuality. They should be taught about date rape, about birth control. They should be taught to assume that anytime they have sex they are risking—boys and girls—AIDS, sexually transmitted disease, and becoming a parent. At this point, when you simply tell them they should "just say no," they look out the window and start singing. It's too little too late.

There should be a marriage between schools and public health. We should have health education programs in schools.

What about the charge that teaching teens about sexuality actually increases sexual activity?

There has never, never been any study that has documented that teaching young people about sex increases sexual activity, and most studies say it decreases sexual activity. In fact, according to a new study ["Impact of High School Condom Availability Program on Sexual Attitudes and Behaviors," *Family Planning Perspectives*, March-April, 1998] even when condoms were made available in a high school, sexual activity did not increase.

How serious are teen pregnancy, STDs and HIV among teens?

There are more than 3 million STDs a year reported in those under 19 years of age. Genital herpes—which cannot be cured—has increased almost 30% in young people in the last eight or nine years. The pregnancy rate is slightly down, but there are still almost 900,000 teen pregnancies a year. When it comes to HIV, the largest increase in cases is seen in teenagers. This is serious. The stakes are very high.

Yet, sex education has been part of the curriculum in many schools for many years. Why isn't it working?

We've not had comprehensive K–12 sexuality education. We're still out there giving kids an annual AIDS lecture. We might as well keep that. We don't teach math by giving one lecture a year. You have to do it all the time and keep reinforcing it. We're not making a committed effort to change things. What we're doing is criticizing and blaming. The problem is, we're willing to sacrifice our children to preserve our Victorian attitudes. We know what to do. We know how to do it. We just don't have the will to get it done.

In the 1960s, when we found out our children were behind in math and science, we added courses in math and science. So if we want to address the social problems our children are having now, we have to put in the programs to do it.

How should a school administrator respond if a parent or group of parents demands that an abstinence-only curriculum be taught?

A superintendent should agree with the parents and put in an abstinence-only program for kindergarten and elementary students. When it comes to older students, he really needs to tell other parents what's going on so they can rise up and fight. Ultimately, a superintendent has to do what his board members tell him to do. But it's the parents who carry the big stick. Parents can get anything they want, and two major studies have shown that most parents want comprehensive sexuality education, with condom availability, in the schools. Yet, because of their silence, they let this other side get their way and destroy their children.

What is the relationship between public health departments, public schools, and the U.S. Surgeon General's office?

There should be a marriage between schools and public health. We should have health education programs in schools along with school-based clinics that would be easily accessible to students and affordable. Now, many young people don't know where to go or don't have the money to pay for health services. We also need to teach people how to be healthy. We have a health-illiterate society, and one place to correct that is in the schools. I think the Surgeon General has a role to play in promoting good health practices and focusing on prevention—to try and make this country as healthy as it can be.

2

Sex Education Should be Taught Primarily by Parents

John F. McCarthy

John F. McCarthy is a monsignor in the Roman Catholic Church.

A 1995 document released by the Roman Catholic Church recognizes the right and duty of parents to teach their children about sex. Schools may assist parents in educating their children, but the primary responsibility for teaching them lies with the parents. The explicit sex education that is taught in the schools corrupts the innocence and purity of young children. Sex education should not include erotic imagery or immoral ideology that would cause a child to think unpure thoughts; it should develop the virtue of chastity in a child.

In *The Truth and Meaning of Human Sexuality* (dated Dec. 8th), published Dec. 20th, 1995, the Pontifical Council for the Family has "blown the whistle" on the imposition of detailed and explicit sex education upon children and adolescents outside of the home. Documents of the Church both past and present have consistently affirmed that the forming and informing of the sexual attitudes of children belongs by right to their parents, but this truth has been violated with increasing frequency in our time by professional educators and others. Now the Council for the Family has placed a note of finality on the issue and has directly called upon parents everywhere to take in hand the right and responsibility that is theirs. (Since the English-language edition of the document was not available until Jan. 15th, 1996, the quotations from the document are my translation from the Italian published text.) While "sex education" in the sense of the cultivation in students of growth toward chaste manhood and womanhood through instruction in the moral teachings of the Church remains, as always, a function of Catholic classrooms, the new document virtually excludes classroom "sex education" in the sense of the presentation of intimate details and aspects of genital behavior and entirely excludes any material that is apt to raise erotic images in the minds of the students.

Reprinted from John F. McCarthy, "On Human Sexuality: A Response of the Holy See to Parents," *The Wanderer*, February 1, 1996, by permission of *The Wanderer*.

The right and duty of parents

The proclamation that the sexual education of children is the right and duty of parents and is to be given by the parents in the atmosphere of the home should not have come as a surprise to anyone. Yet it has come as a surprise to many. On this crucial issue, genuine confusion had arisen in the Church because of a misreading of what Vatican Council II proclaimed in its Declaration on Christian Education *(Gravissimum Educationis,* n. 1). The Second Vatican Council declared that "as they grow older, they [children and young people] should receive a positive and prudent education in matters relating to sex," and from this pronouncement many educators and others came to believe that Vatican II had mandated what Pope Pius XI had earlier condemned, namely, that children and young people should be instructed in the classroom about the details of human genital activity. Now the Pontifical Council for the Family has brought out a lengthy treatise and guide for parents in which it is made abundantly clear that the taking over of the sexual education of children by the schools is not what the Second Vatican Council meant by this pronouncement.

As this new document points out: "The Church has always affirmed that the parents have the duty and the right to be the first and principal educators of their children" (n. 5). Thus, canon 793.1 of the 1983 revised Code of Canon Law affirms: "Parents, and those who take their place, have both the obligation and the right to educate their children. Catholic parents have also the duty and the right to choose those means and institutes which, in their local circumstances, can best promote the Catholic education of their children." Canon 796.2 goes on to say: "There must be the closest cooperation between parents and the teachers to whom they entrust their children to be educated. In fulfilling their task, teachers are to collaborate closely with the parents and willingly listen to them; associations and meetings of parents are to be set up and held in high esteem." Again, canon 798 states the rule: "Parents are to send their children to those schools which will provide for their Catholic education. If they cannot do this, they are bound to ensure the proper Catholic education of their children outside the school."

The forming and informing of the sexual attitudes of children belongs by right to their parents.

The Second Vatican Council, in its Declaration on Christian Education (n. 3), presents the same basic truth: "As it is the parents who have given life to their children, on them lies the greatest obligation of educating their family. They must therefore be recognized as being primarily and principally responsible for their education. The role of parents in education is of such importance that it is almost impossible to provide an adequate substitute." The Second Vatican Council here refers the reader to Pope Pius XI's encyclical *On the Christian Education of Youth (Divini Illius Magistri, AAS 22* [1930], p. 50 ff.), and to two declarations of Pope Pius XII.

In narrating the truth about human sexuality, the newly published document of the Council for the Family (nn. 41–42) refers parents to this declaration of Vatican Council II, restated by Pope John Paul II in *Familiaris Consortio* (1981): "The right and duty of parents to give education is *essential,* since it is connected with the transmission of human life; it is *original and primary* with regard to the educational role of others, on account of the uniqueness of the living relationship between parents and children; and it is *irreplaceable and inalienable,* and therefore incapable of being entirely delegated to others or usurped by others" (n. 36). This right and duty of parents is expressed also in the *Charter of the Rights of the Family* (art. 5) and in *The Catechism of the Catholic Church* (n. 2221 ff.).

The problem treated in the present document is the widespread usurpation, especially by professional educators and by the mass media, of the right of parents to educate their children in matters relating to human sexuality. In times past, when explicit sexual education was not customary, the children were objectively protected by the values implanted in the surrounding culture, but now no longer, and the truth about man has been obscured by such things as the "trivializing of sex." The mass media invade homes with "depersonalized information" for which young persons are not prepared, in a context "devoid of values based upon life, human love, and the family." Schools have undertaken programs of sex education in place of the family, "usually with the goal of information alone," sometimes resulting in a "real deformation of consciences." In this situation, says the Council for the Family, "many Catholic parents have turned to the Church to take up the burden by offering guidance and suggestions for the education of their children," pointing out "their difficulties in the face of teaching given in the school and then brought home by the children." Thus, this guide for parents has been issued in response to their "repeated and urgent requests" (all stated in n. 1).

The same document of the Council for the Family goes on to stress the right and duty of parents to form their children in chaste love (n. 41), basing its position upon the following teaching of Pope John Paul II:

> The educational service of parents must aim firmly at a training in the area of sex which is truly and fully personal: For sexuality is an enrichment of the whole person—body, emotions, and soul—and it manifests its inmost meaning in leading the person to the gift of self in love. Sex education, which is a basic right and duty of parents, must always be carried out under their attentive guidance, whether at home or in educational centers chosen and controlled by them. In this regard, the Church reaffirms the law of subsidiarity, which the school is bound to observe when it cooperates in sex education, by entering into the same spirit that animates the parents. In this context *education for chastity* is absolutely essential, for it is a virtue that develops a person's authentic maturity and makes him or her capable of respecting and fostering the 'nuptial meaning' of the body. Indeed, Christian parents, discerning the signs of God's call, will devote special attention and care to education in virginity or celibacy as the supreme form of that self-giving that constitutes the very meaning of human sexuality. In

view of the close links between the sexual dimension of the person and his or her ethical values, education must bring the children to a knowledge of and respect for the moral norms as the necessary and highly valuable guarantee for responsible personal growth in human sexuality. For this reason, the Church is firmly opposed to an often widespread form of imparting sex information dissociated from moral principles. That would merely be an introduction to the experience of pleasure and a stimulus leading to the loss of serenity—while still in the years of innocence—by opening the way to vice (*Familiaris Consortio,* n. 37).

The document of the Council for the Family bemoans, with Pope John Paul II, "certain programs of sex education introduced into the schools, often notwithstanding the contrary opinion and even protests of many parents" (n. 24). The primary task of the family carries with it for parents the right that their children not be obliged at school to take part in courses regarding sexual life which are not in accord with their own religious and moral convictions (n. 49). The document recommends to parents that they follow attentively every kind of sexual education that is given to their children outside of the home and that they withdraw them whenever this does not correspond with their own principles (n. 117).

The document allows that there are various ways in which professional educators can assist parents in this task, but "such assistance never means taking away from the parents or diminishing their formative right and duty," because this remains "original and primary," "irreplaceable and inalienable." In keeping with the principle of subsidiarity and, therefore, with due subordination and in the proper order of things, educators and others outside of the home may assist parents in their task of sexual education, but "it is clear that the assistance of others must be given chiefly to the parents rather than to the children" (n. 145).

Against classroom sex education

The classic warning against harmful and inopportune classroom sex education is that given by Pope Pius XI on Dec. 31st, 1929, in his great encyclical *On the Christian Education of Youth:*

> Another very grave danger is that naturalism which nowadays invades the field of education in that most delicate matter of purity of morals. Far too common is the error of those who with dangerous assurance and under an ugly term propagate a so-called sex education, falsely imagining they can forearm youth against the dangers of sensuality by means purely natural, such as a foolhardy initiation and precautionary instruction for all indiscriminately, even in public; and, worse still, by exposing them at an early age to the occasions, in order to accustom them, so it is argued, and as it were to harden them against such dangers.
>
> Such persons grievously err in refusing to recognize the inborn weakness of human nature and the law of mind *(Rom.*

7:23), and also in ignoring the experience of facts, from which it is clear that, particularly in young people, evil practices are the effect not so much of ignorance of intellect as of weakness of a will exposed to dangerous occasions, and unsupported by the means of grace.

In this extremely delicate matter, if, all things considered, some private instruction is found necessary and opportune from those who hold from God the commission to teach and have the grace of state, every precaution must be taken. Such precautions are well known in traditional Christian education and are described adequately by Antoniano cited above, when he says:

"Such is our misery and inclination to sin, that often in the very things considered to be remedies against sin, we find occasions for and inducements to sin itself. Hence it is of the highest importance that a good father, while discussing with his son a matter so delicate, should be well on his guard and not descend to details, nor refer to the various ways in which this infernal hydra destroys with its poison so large a portion of the world; otherwise it may happen that instead of extinguishing this fire, he unwittingly stirs or kindles it in the simple and tender heart of the child. Speaking generally, during the period of childhood it suffices to employ those remedies which produce the double effect of opening the door to the virtue of purity and closing the door upon vice" (*Divini Illius Magistri*, nn. 65–67).

Because the Second Vatican Council called for a "positive and prudent *education* in matters relating to sex," many educators came to believe that this was a mandate for the inclusion of courses regarding human genital behavior in the academic programs of the schools, but the teaching of the Universal Church even since the Second Vatican Council has been that the parents are the prime *educators* of their children, so that Vatican II was simply calling upon parents to recognize their duty in this regard. The present document of the Council for the Family speaks directly to parents to encourage them in this task, following the lead of Pope John Paul II. While Pope Pius XI and Pope Pius XII laid some stress upon the discreet and opportune instruction of their children by parents in the home, Vatican II saw a stronger need because of the growing attacks upon the chastity of children from sources outside of the home, and thus it saw a greater need for parents to intervene.

This instruction of the Council for the Family has been issued to make parents aware of the "sexual revolution" that since the 1960s has been militating against the responsible use of sexuality in the family while promoting an alleged right to sexual pleasure for its own sake. Alfonso Cardinal Lopez Trujillo, president of the Pontifical Council for the Family, announcing the document in an article in the daily edition of *L'Osservatore Romano* (Dec. 21st, 1995), says that the "sexual revolution" is aimed at the separation of the sexual act from its true meaning, even on the part of married couples, and thus fosters a betrayal of spousal love.

Countless young people, he says, have been swept away by this avalanche of unbridled pleasure. The effect of this revolution has been that human society is becoming constantly more "eroticized." He notes that "scientific research itself has become the slave of industry to serve, with the successes of its investigations, a commercial view of life in which profit seems to be the only real purpose, and this is placed above the good of persons and of society." The sexual revolution "was pushed forward and accelerated by new scientific discoveries, in particular that of the [abortifacient] 'pill'." And so, he adds, "the opulent society, driven by the euphoria of hedonism, has offered, outside of the family and with an outlook not inspired for the good of the person but for the consumption of goods, the sex market and sex as theater and pastime (*loisir*)."

The primary task of the family carries with it for parents the right that their children not be obliged at school to take part in courses regarding sexual life which are not in accord with their own religious and moral convictions.

From the above-cited passage it is clear what kind of "sex education" was excluded by Pope Pius XI, namely: a) recourse to merely natural means with no attention to the supernatural order of things or the actual condition of fallen and redeemed mankind; b) foolhardy initiation and precautionary instruction for all indiscriminately even in public; c) exposing children to the occasions of sin with the pretext of "hardening them" against dangers; d) overlooking the weakness of will that children normally have; e) descent into details with the danger of enkindling lust in the simple and tender heart of the child. In describing "the situation today" (1983), the Sacred Congregation for Catholic Education, in its instruction entitled *Educational Guidance in Human Love* (pp. 5–6), points out that this teaching of Pope Pius XI declared "information of a naturalist character, precociously and indiscriminately imparted," to be wrong and harmful. Developments of the idea of "individual, positive sex education" before Vatican II never challenged this teaching and always considered such education to be "within the ambit of the family" (*Ibid.*). But because *Familiaris Consortio* in 1981 and *Educational Guidance in Human Love* in 1983 spoke of the role of "educational centers" and the task of "the school" with regard to sex education, many educators came erroneously to believe that for practical purposes the initiative in the sexual formation of children was being transferred from the parents to the school. To recognize this error more completely, it is useful to consider the role of the school in the moral formation of children and the meaning of the expression "sex education."

The role of the school

Pope Pius XI, in his encyclical *On the Christian Education of Youth*, points out that "education belongs pre-eminently to the Church" (n. 15). Hence, the Church has a right "to decide what may help or harm Christian education" (n. 18). Thus, he says, "the mission of education regards before all, above all, primarily, the Church and the family, and this by natural and divine law" (n. 40). In fact, it is "the inalienable right as well as the indispensable duty of the Church to watch over the entire education of her children, in all institutions, public or private . . . insofar as religion and morality are concerned" (n. 23). But the "first natural and necessary element" in the educational environment of the child "is the family" (n. 71). For this reason, Pope Pius XI calls the attention of bishops and others to "the present-day lamentable decline in family education" (n. 73) and he implores "pastors of souls, by every means in their power, by instructions and catechisms, by word of mouth and written articles widely distributed, to warn Christian parents of their grave obligations," not just in general, but "with practical and specific application to the various responsibilities of parents touching the religious, moral, and civil training of their children" (n. 74). "Let it be borne in mind," he says, that since the school is "an institution subsidiary and complementary to the family and the Church," it follows logically that "it must not be in opposition to, but in positive accord with those other two elements, and form with them a perfect moral union, constituting one sanctuary of education, as it were, with the family and the Church. Otherwise, it is doomed to fail of its purpose, and to become instead an agent of destruction" (n. 77).

In the light of these distinctions it becomes clear that *Educational Guidance in Human Love* did not advocate the transfer of information about human genital behavior from the family to the classroom; it simply gave advice as to how parents as educators in sexuality can better form their children and how professional teachers can assist parents in the general area of character formation. Thus, what the Sacred Congregation for Catholic Education actually said in *Educational Guidance in Human Love* is that "the role of the school should be that of assisting and completing the work of parents, furnishing children and adolescents with an evaluation of 'sexuality as value and task of the whole person, created male and female in the image of God'" (n. 69, quoting *Familiaris Consortio*, n. 32). Here, then, what is directly in focus is "the whole person," not genital behavior as a supposed subject in itself.

The role of the school should be that of assisting and completing the work of parents.

To clarify this, *Educational Guidance in Human Love* also says (again quoting from *Familiaris Consortio*) that "sex education, which is a basic right and duty of parents, must also be carried out under their attentive guidance" according to "the law of subsidiarity, which the school is bound to observe when it cooperates in sex education, by entering into the same spirit that animates the parents" (n. 17). It says that "education, in the first place, is the duty of the family," which is "the best environment to accomplish the obligation of securing a gradual education in sexual life" (n. 48). It also declares that "with regard to the more intimate aspects, whether biological or affective, an individual education should be bestowed, preferably within the sphere of the family" (n. 58). Only, then, "if parents do not feel able to perform this duty, may they have recourse to others who enjoy their confidence" (n. 59). Where the school is called upon to intervene in matters relating to sexuality, "individual [not class-room] sex education always retains prior value and cannot be entrusted indiscriminately to just any member of the school community," but "re-quires from the teacher outstanding sensitivity in initiating the child and adolescent in the problems of love and life without disturbing their psy-chological development" (n. 71). Groups, and above all mixed groups, "require special precautions," so that, "in each case, the responsible au-thorities must examine with parents the propriety of proceeding in such a manner" (n. 72).

The Truth and Meaning of Human Sexuality applies these principles by declaring that the school should not require pupils to assist at courses which are not in accord with "the religious and moral convictions of their parents" (n. 64). It advises parents to withdraw their children from every form of sex education given in the school which "does not correspond to their own principles" (n. 117). It forbids the school to penalize the child or his family for exercising the right to withdraw from undesired instruc-tion about human sexuality (n. 120). A fact that is clear from these vari-ous principles is that no such instruction should be undertaken by the school without the specific authorization of the parents. The permission of parents may not be presumed; rather, authorization should be ex-pressly given by the parents for each child involved.

Since the proper order is not Church, school, family, but Church, family, school, we can be grateful to the Council for the Family for call-ing this fact to the attention of parents and for calling upon bishops' con-ferences, clergy, and religious to assist and encourage parents to give a proper "sex education" to their children within the sanctuary of the home (nn. 147–148). But what does the word "sex" mean in the expres-sion "sex education"?

The meaning of sex education

It is important to realize that the most common meaning of the word "sex" has changed drastically since the beginning of this century. "Hav-ing sex" is now taken to mean, not "being male or female," but "having genital intercourse." Thus "sex education" comes to mean "learning about genital intercourse" apart from its context in the human vocation and in the moral realities which should surround it. Such was the inten-tion of the secular humanist originators of the term "sex education." By placing the focus of attention exclusively upon the material act of geni-tal intercourse, "sex educators" not only separate the mind of the child from the familial context of this act, but they also cut the child off from a full understanding of his or her own psychological makeup. When Pope Pius XI, in Divini Illius Magistri (quoted above), speaks of those who prop-agate "under an ugly term" a so-called sex education, it is to this false meaning of the word "sex" that he is alluding. The words "sex" and "sex-ual," taken in their proper sense, are not ugly terms, but what is ugly is the impurity associated with the erotic imagery and immoral ideology of the "sex education" originally devised by secular humanists and still in use. It is this corrupting imagery and ideology that functions today in most "sex education" classes. Hence, Cardinal Lopez Trujillo, in his announcing article, warns parents that "the 'sex' education being presented is devoid, most of the time, of a true concept of sexuality." When Church documents from the time of the Second Vatican Council speak of a "positive and prudent sex education," they mean formation into full manhood and womanhood, without an inordinate focus upon the genital and the erotic, but in the joy and warmth of the virtue of chastity. This is explained at length in *The Truth and Meaning of Human Sexuality*. Sex education, in the morally acceptable sense of that term, is "formation in chastity" and is inseparable from the cultivation of all the other virtues, especially of that Christian love called *charity* (n. 55). Formation in chastity aims at three objectives: "a) to preserve in the family a positive atmosphere of love, of virtue and of respect for the gifts of God, in particular for the gift of life; b) to help children gradually to understand the value of sexuality and of chastity by supporting their growth with enlightenment, example, and prayer; c) to help them to understand and to discover their own vocation to matrimony or to consecrated virginity for the Kingdom of Heaven in harmony with and in respect for their aptitudes, inclinations, and gifts of the Spirit" (n. 22).

Regarding the manner of instructing their children at the proper time in sexual matters of an intimate nature, the guide for parents cautions parents against being either too explicit or too vague (n. 75) and to refrain from discussing deviant sexual practices where there is no special need (n. 125).

Advice to parents

The first basic rule for a positive approach given to parents in the new document (n. 122) is that "human sexuality is a sacred mystery which must be presented in accordance with the doctrinal and moral teaching of the Church, always taking into account the effects of original sin." It is obvious that most public schools fail to respect this rule and even systematically violate it. But even many Church schools are flagrant offenders. The open dissent of many teachers in Catholic schools to the doctrinal and moral teachings of the Church is proof enough, apart from the twisted notion of sexuality that has invaded Catholic intellectual circles. Witness to this tragedy is the report *Human Sexuality* published under the auspices of the Catholic Theological Society of America (Paramus, N.J.: Paulist Press, 1977).

The CTSA report proclaimed to Catholic educators a long series of morally irresponsible, shocking, and pastorally devastating "conclusions," such as the following: a) that Sacred Scripture does not necessarily forbid any form of genital behavior whatsoever (p. 31), b) that adultery can be morally acceptable (p. 15); c) that contraception can be wholesome and moral (p. 122); d) that premarital intercourse can be a morally good experience (pp. 155–158); e) that evaluations of premarital intercourse that are "sin-centered" should be avoided (pp. 173–174); f) that obscene words are now part of the common vocabulary and may be used in polite conversation (p. 235); g) that pornographic material is not immoral (p. 236); h) that masturbation is not sinful (p. 220); i) that homosexual intercourse is not wrong in itself (p. 198); j) that deviant sexual practices are not evil (p. 77); k) that prostitution is not sinful in itself (pp. 16, 30–31, 96); l) that, until Church and state change their laws to accommodate the conclusions of this report, people should just "proceed discreetly with their own sexual project" (p 56); m) that sex education in keeping with the views expressed in this report should be made to permeate all areas of educational development (p. 237).

What sensible parents would entrust their children to sex educators like this? It is no wonder that the Council for the Family now advises parents to beware of "professional associations of sex educators, sex counselors, and sex therapists, because their work is often based upon unsound theories, devoid of scientific value, and closed to an authentic anthropology, which do not recognize the true value of chastity" (n. 138).

Sex education, in the morally acceptable sense of that term, is "formation in chastity" and is inseparable from the cultivation of all the other virtues.

In addition to all anti-life indoctrination (nn. 135–139), any material or approach that excites the prurient interest of children or fails to alert them to the effects of original sin is excluded by the new document (nn. 122–123). Any material, we might say, that causes children to fantasize sexual intercourse would place them in a proximate occasion of consenting to impure thoughts. "No material which is by nature erotic should ever be presented to children or young people of any age, whether individually or in groups. This *principle of decency* is needed to safeguard the virtue of chastity" (n. 126).

Thus, the new document, in addition to excluding any system of education which prescinds from the true nature of man, as known from reason and Revelation, or which presents erotic experience as an end in itself, also rejects the indiscreet presentation of material in the classroom. Even in Catholic schools (which are not taken up specifically in the document) the same dangers are present, in some ways to an even greater degree inasmuch as teachers in Catholic schools who violate these norms are not only in effect propagating the spirit of the world, the flesh, and the Devil, but doing so with the apparent blessing of the Church. In some textbooks which present material bordering on the prurient, the inclusion of some Catholic dogmatic and moral principles does not compensate for the rupturing of a chaste academic atmosphere and of a sense of propriety among the pupils.

Cardinal Lopez Trujillo, in his announcing article, avers that the spread of AIDS "suggests to many 'experts,' paradoxically, not the need of temperance and self-control, but access to another market, that of 'free and safe sex,' where true freedom and security fail." Thus, public authorities have favored AIDS education in the schools by way of information "reduced to a weak and exclusively hygienic view," without any framework of values. He notes that this revolutionary idea of human sexuality has given rise to the inhuman "separation of sexuality from matrimony and from the family, of love from life within matrimony, of the unitive from the procreative aspect of the conjugal act, giving great support to campaigns in favor of abortion, contraception, and 'family planning'." This suggests a further example. Everyone knows that AIDS is spread, not only by sexual intercourse, but also by the use of infected hypodermic needles, especially by users of narcotics. Why aren't children in public schools being taught the safe use of hypodermic needles? Why aren't clean syringes being made freely available in schools, dormitories, and other gathering places? Is it not because the damage to children induced toward the use of narcotics constitutes a greater physical and psychological evil than the good which is hoped for? That leads us to suspect the hypocrisy of "safe-sex" educators who refuse to admit the psychological and spiritual damage inflicted upon persons induced to extramarital sexual intercourse.

The document points out that other educators may help parents, but not substitute themselves for the parents, "if not for serious reasons of physical or moral incapacity" (n. 23). It seems clear that "moral incapacity" would include culpable indifference of parents to the educational needs of their children or the intention to corrupt their children rather than to form them in chaste love (cf. n. 118). In this case, there are reasons for conscientious outsiders to provide certain needed information to neglected children, but there are no good reasons for invading the chaste atmosphere of good families with unwanted sex education, even if it does not offend against Catholic doctrine, and it also appears to be a crime and a scandal to taint the sober academic atmosphere of any classroom with sexual language and ideas that a child should not hear even in the street. What parents are facing is a tidal wave of sexual hedonism that has swept over civil society, and from civil society into the classroom, and from the classroom into their families.

There are no good reasons for invading the chaste atmosphere of good families with unwanted sex education.

In *Familiaris Consortio* (n. 40), Pope John Paul II points out the duty of parents "to commit themselves totally to a cordial and active relationship with the teachers and the school authorities," while, at the same time, "if ideologies opposed to the Christian faith are taught in the schools, the family must join with other families, if possible through family associations, and with all its strength and with wisdom help the young not to depart from the faith." *The Truth and Meaning of Human Sexuality* invites parents to form associations, where necessary or useful, in order to carry out an education of their children "marked with the true values of the person and of Christian love, taking a clear stand that rises above ethical utilitarianism" (n. 24). The document urges parents to join together also "to oppose injurious forms of sex education and to make sure that their children are educated according to Christian principles and in a manner consonant with their personal development" (n. 114).

The new document is clear in inviting parents to prepare themselves adequately to give the needed instruction, and in suggesting that the more capable parents help the others in the preparation of textbooks and other materials that might be used (n. 147). Due emphasis is also given (n. 118) to the right of the child to be able to live his or her sexuality and to grow in it "in conformity with Christian principles, and, thus, to exercise also the virtue of chastity" to the extent that "no educator—not even the parents—may interfere with this right." The child has a right "to be informed in a timely manner by his own parents about moral and sexual questions in such a manner as to reinforce his desire to be chaste and to be formed in chastity" (n. 119).

The Church's beliefs

Concluding observations. a) The Church has a mission to promote the doctrinal and moral formation of the human race. Schools, and especially Catholic schools, assist the hierarchy in this apostolate, and they also assist parents, who have the prior right and duty to instruct their children in faith and morals. Schools which have been entrusted by parents with the academic formation of their children have a strict obligation to present the full and unadulterated dogmatic and moral teaching of the Church. Where schools fail in this obligation, parents have a duty to protect the faith of their children, by individual action and even, "if possible, through family associations" (*Familiaris Consortio,* n. 40).

b) Catholic schools have a mission to assist parents in the intellectual and moral education of their children, and parents have a duty to give full cooperation to the schools they choose. But schools do not have a mission to teach children the intimate details of sexual behavior. Where parents are demonstrably culpable in not giving the proper instruction to their children, the school may have a role, but the classroom is usually not the place. Basically, it is the role of the school to provide the intellectual and moral framework whereby the child can make proper moral decisions. The image of sexual intercourse is not an academic subject; it is an image which has moral meaning in the context of a proper mental framework, but which is the essence of impure thinking when focused upon outside a framework that gives it rationality. Sex education, as it was conceived originally by secular hedonists, is a movement to corrupt the minds of children with impure thoughts by forcing them to visualize genital intercourse, natural and unnatural, without there being any real pedagogical need for them to visualize this. Moral theologians have always taught that to watch sexual intercourse is an immediate occasion of mortal sin, and this includes watching it in a graphic drawing or in the fantasy of one's own imagination.

The image of natural sexual intercourse is morally good in the framework of marital intent. It should not be dwelt upon directly and explicitly outside of the context of matrimony. Images of unnatural sexual intercourse are particularly damaging to the minds of the young. It so happens that, in some large libraries, books describing deviant sexual behavior (including homosexual intercourse) are locked in a special room and can be viewed only by qualified specialists. The reason is that reading about such activity is extremely prurient and has no proportionate academic value. It can simply cause disturbing mental images that may remain for a long time. Yet there are many sex education courses in which these prurient unnatural images are raised in class. The only way that these images can be controlled while they are being considered is in an adult framework such as that of medicine, clinical psychology, law, or criminology. They do not belong in a high school.

c) The "formation in chastity" recommended by the teachings of the Popes and of the Holy See does not mean classroom courses about genital activity with material added relating to the virtue of chastity. Intimate details about genital behavior belong in short discussions on an individual basis, usually with a parent. The new document (n. 133) advises parents to monitor courses and study aids to make sure that all potentially erotic or overly detailed material has been eliminated. The school has an obligation to drop any material to which the parents object. The parents do not need to convince the school authorities that their objections are valid; it is rather the school authorities who need to convince the parents that contested material is not objectionable.

d) This new document on formation in chastity calls upon episcopal conferences to assist parents to teach their children at home (n. 147). While bishops have consistently assisted Catholic schools to operate, it seems clear that insufficient attention has been given to helping parents to home-school their children, even in localities where no Catholic school is available. A massive effort of assistance to parents by bishops is now needed. An immediate beginning could be made by the republication of this new document of the Holy See in every diocesan newspaper, or by making the booklet available to every family in every diocese. The document invites the clergy to take sides with the parents in conflicts with schools over the violation of their parental right to safeguard the chastity of their children (n. 148). Let good parents proceed unmolested to form in their children a healthy aversion for sins of impurity, and let modern technology undertake a search for a "prophylactic device" that will block the transmission of improper sex educational material, so that hedonistic sex educators will be able to proclaim the "sexual revolution" to their heart's content without infecting with the virus of impurity the minds of the children who happen to compose their captive audiences.

3

Sex Education Should Emphasize Values

Amitai Etzioni

Amitai Etzioni is a professor at George Washington University, founder and chair of the Communitarian Network, and editor of the quarterly communitarian journal Responsive Community.

Sex education should include more than a lesson in human biology and hygiene. Students should be urged to defer both sex and marriage until they are mature enough to handle the responsibilities and self-control required of sexual intimacy. However, teens should be provided with the information necessary to protect themselves against disease and pregnancy should they decide not to wait. Most importantly, parents should be involved in their children's sex-education programs.

Instead of approaching the discussion of sex in public schools as a matter of health and safety bereft of moral content or forbidding discussion of sex out of traditional moral concerns (seeking to rely exclusively on the family and religious institutions for this purpose), schools should develop a program of education that provides children with the facts they need to know, within the context of values that responsible and moral persons seek to affirm and embody in their lives. Sex education should not be taught as a chapter in human hygiene or human biology, akin to dental care or car mechanics. We can find better sources and role models for teaching this subject than what the birds and the bees do. Nor should sex education be treated as if it is, was, or could be, value-free.

What should be included

Education for interpersonal relations, family life, and intimacy should occur in all public schools, at least in junior high schools (or middle schools) and high schools. The program should include discussion of human nature, an examination of human beings as social creatures who require one another; who find deep satisfaction, longer and healthier lives,

Reprinted, with permission, from Amitai Etzioni, "Education for Intimacy," *Tikkun Magazine: A Bimonthly Jewish Critique of Politics, Culture, and Society*, March/April 1997. Information and subscriptions are available from *Tikkun*, 26 Fell St., San Francisco, CA 94102.

when they are part of lasting social relations; and who have transcendental needs for meanings and moral values. The program should explore the responsibilities that we have for one another as members of a community, and ways we can strengthen our relations with one another, as co-workers, neighbors, friends and potential family members. This topic includes teaching ways to work out differences, by techniques such as improved communication skills and conflict resolution. Discussion of family life will explore matters such as the nature of the commitments involved in marriage; sharing decision-making in such matters as relocation and forming and adhering to budget; and the issues raised by intimate relations, ranging from the avoidance of exploitative relations to the use of contraceptives.

Schools now cover a good portion of these topics in a variety of classes such as social studies and home economics, while ignoring other parts. Schools need to combine some of these elements already in place with new ones, to provide a comprehensive and morally sound approach to interpersonal relations and to provide the needed context for teaching sex education.

Specifically, a public school program of sex education should be folded into a much more encompassing treatment of interpersonal relations, family life, and intimacy, to be developed by taking into account the premises and principles here articulated.

Developing a strong character needs to be at the core of all education programs, and particularly of programs dedicated to interpersonal relations, family life, and intimacy. Persons of weak character cannot take responsibility for their actions, abide by values they themselves believe in, be good partners in a relationship, or be upstanding members of a community. Character development is essential both because without it, all other educational efforts will be undermined (as we see in disorderly classrooms), and whatever education is imparted will be woefully lacking.

Two personality capabilities stand out as leading the agenda of character building: First, a person of good character is able to restrain his or her raw impulses by channeling them into socially constructive and morally sound avenues rather than mindlessly yielding to them. Such a person can express affection and commitment in socially and morally appropriate manners. Second, a person of good character can empathize with the other person involved who may have different needs or be in a different stage of sexual and social development.

Sex education should not be taught as a chapter in human hygiene or human biology, akin to dental care or car mechanics.

The underlying orientation of the intimacy program to sex is that sex is inherently neither good nor evil, neither pure nor sinful; the context makes all the difference. Sex is somewhat akin to nuclear energy: properly contained it is a boon to the world; let loose it can be a highly destructive force. As Kevin Ryan, professor at the School of Education at Boston University, put it:

"Sex is strong stuff. It is a powerful force in people's lives, and as such, it can be a strong force for individual happiness and family stability. On the other hand, selfish and uncontrolled sex can be a raging cyclone, making havoc of those in its path."

We find throughout history extreme attempts to control sex through barbaric acts such as genital mutilation, stoning of prostitutes and summary executions of adulterous princesses. And we find cultures that seek to "free" sex from its moral and social context, tolerating forcing children to marry old men and accepting child prostitution. The facts that need to be shared with the young generation are, as we learn from both historical and contemporary experiences, that both attempts to repress sex as well as to let it roam freely, cause much human misery.

What girls seek most is information on how to refuse to engage in sexual acts without hurting someone's feelings.

Sexual exploitation, for example, is far from unknown, even in our society. A high proportion of teen pregnancies are caused by men who are not high school boys, but who are at least five years older than the girls they impregnate. Frequently, these are men who hang around the mothers of the girls involved and sex is non-consensual. Seventy-five percent of teenage pregnancies and youth-affected STDs would still occur if all teenage boys refrained from having sex; fifty-one percent of pregnancies in junior high school would still occur if teenage boys refrained from having sex, according to one study. Incest is also all too common. Strategies for dealing with those who pressure children to have sex should be included in all intimacy programs.

Several studies and surveys of teenage girls have found that, more than information about contraception, STDs, HIV, and pregnancy, what girls seek most is information on how to refuse to engage in sexual acts without hurting someone's feelings. Better communication skills are also necessary for boys, particularly relating to rape and sexual harassment prevention, and how to relate better to fellow human beings. These skills make people into better friends, employees, neighbors and community members. They are particularly significant in the context of sex education.

Even much less severe expressions of sex are matters of serious concern. Making sexual advances to someone committed to one's friend is a quick way to lose that friendship and to offend one's community. The same holds for continuing to make sexual advances to those who indicate that they do not appreciate being approached.

In contrast, sex properly contextualized is a precondition of our future. Sex can be an appropriate way to cement relations that have properly matured, and it can be a source of much joy. In short, sex should always be viewed, treated, and taught within the context of values and relations.

Specifically, when the general orientation of the program is brought to bear on sex education, the program should stress that bringing children into the world is a moral act—one that entails a set of personal and social responsibilities. We all need to appreciate that sex is not a merely biological act; sex is much more than "recreational." It is an act that can carry with it serious consequences including loss of life. Responsible persons weigh the moral issues involved; they take into account that yielding to impulse in this area can lead to dire consequences for the child to be born, restrict the life chances of the parents, and corrode the values of the communities in which we are all members.

Education for intimacy seeks to encourage children to refrain from having children. Children born to children often suffer considerably physiologically, psychologically, and otherwise. These babies are more prone to illnesses, anxieties, and other afflictions. They often become public charges in a society that is increasingly disinclined to attend to children properly.

Children who have babies often find their life opportunities seriously constricted. They are much less likely to complete their studies, find work, and otherwise develop their own life, economically, socially and otherwise.

When educational programs favor that young people defer engaging in sex, the question is raised, should sex be deferred until a person is 18? 21? married? The question is often raised by those who argue that sex is only proper within marriage. While much is to be said for deferring sex until two people have made the kind of permanent commitment and mutual responsibility implied by marriage, marriage does not provide the only criterion. We would urge young teens to defer both sex and marriage on the grounds that they are likely not to be ready to make a responsible decision in either department. And we are less troubled by intimate relations between mature adults than between children. Maturity is measured by behavior rather than chronological age, but it is more common among those who are older than those who are younger.

How sex education should be taught

Many discussions of sex education start with the question of which sex education methodology to follow. I deliberately delayed addressing this issue to emphasize that if proper values and interpersonal skill development are included in the intimacy education program, intercourse is no longer the only issue or main focus. At the same time we maintain that programs that deal only with values or relations but exclude specific sex education are insufficient for reasons that will become evident shortly.

Sex should always be viewed, treated, and taught within the context of values and relations.

The methodology I favor diverges from the notion that sex should be described simply as a natural, healthy act and that children should be taught how to proceed safely, but not be discouraged otherwise. Statements such as "sexuality is a natural and healthy part of living" and "all persons are sexual" may be correct by some standards of psychiatry (which consider all erotic responses sexual) but are open to gross misinterpretation when given to children, especially without the proper normative context. To state that "the primary goal of sexuality education is the promotion of sexual health" is particularly unfortunate in this context. At the same time, approaches which treat sex not tied to procreation as sinful, shameful, or dirty should be avoided. To say, in this context, that "most merciful God, we confess we are in bondage to sin and cannot free ourselves," may speak to some people with religious commitments (but surely offends others); provided as a part of a statement about "human sexuality" it sends a rather different message than the one endorsed here.

Merely relying on willpower, "just say no," is psychologically naive and unrealistic.

Sex should be viewed originally as a primordial urge. Like all others, it cannot be ignored and should not be suppressed but its expressions must be subject to self-control. What is needed is (a) that a person will form judgments before he or she acts and (b) that a person will channel expression of this urge into morally and socially proper, responsible channels.

Narrow sex education programs that favor sharing full information about safe sex with young children are problematic. These programs tend to assume that the resulting effects of encouraging sexual activity are minimal. Also troublesome are programs that address contraception in what Jane Mauldon and Kristin Luker say is ". . . a tone of value neutrality, focusing on clinical information to the exclusion of social, emotional, and moral aspects of sex," as some do.

Abstinence-only programs

At the same time I am also concerned about programs that promote abstinence only and do not take sufficiently into account the moral issues that arise by the many (even those in highly religious groups) who do not adhere to the high standards involved, by engaging in sex, and hence risking exposure to AIDS and other STDs, or experience unwanted pregnancies. These effects can be significantly reduced, albeit not eliminated, if students are taught about safer sex.

Educators, parents, community members and policy-makers need to understand that there are ways to strongly urge young people to defer sexual behavior and still provide information for those who proceed anyhow, without making these two messages cancel each other out or seem contradictory. Schools ought to employ programs that urge children to wait—at least until they are mature enough to deal with the consequences of their sexual acts—but also provide them with information on how to conduct themselves if they do not wait. Responsibility should include the notion of deferring sex and engaging in it in a responsible manner. This position is advocated by Bishop Albert Rouet, the chairman of the French Roman Catholic bishops' social committee, among others.

In dealing with other topics, divorce for instance, religious groups have found ways to extol the importance of preserving marriage, and still counsel those who divorce. The same can be done for sex education. One can strongly advocate abstinence, but also provide youngsters with age-appropriate sex information and ways to proceed responsibly and more safely, lest they rely on misconstrued notions provided by much less wholesome and irresponsible sources. (This approach is sometimes referred to as "abstinence, plus.")

A naive and unrealistic theory

Merely relying on willpower, "just say no," is psychologically naive and unrealistic. Educators should point out that (a) use of drugs and alcohol reduces our self-control; and that (b) other forms of intimacy than intercourse are also best deferred. Our grandparents had a point: Dressing eight-year-old girls with training bras, arranging "socials" with close dancing for nine-year-old children, and other such activities do not always lead to premature sexual experimentation but neither are they without any such effects.

Children need to be taught that the use of alcohol and drugs lowers a person's ability to deal with urges in ways that are socially constructive and morally responsible. They need to learn—and above all experience— the joy of living up to their moral values and social commitment by engaging in acts such as community service, peer mentoring, sports, successful completion of taxing assignments and sharing in the household duties. "Just say no" should be preceded, accompanied and followed by mores one finds reason or value for saying "yes" to. The sociological record shows that those positively engaged, are most able to resist yielding to their raw impulses. There are so many other meaningful and enjoyable activities to cultivate.

The program envisioned should not be limited to lectures and reading material. Role playing, role modeling, peer mentoring, school assemblies, plays, tapes and other educational techniques should be used. Acquiring communication skills allows people to fend off unwanted and premature sexual advances without feeling inadequate, guilty, or isolated. They enable youngsters to handle conflicts that arise when the pace of development of two or more young people varies. Assemblies, peer juries, and other such educational techniques help develop the moral voice of the school community.

Parents should be involved; they have both rights and responsibilities in this area. If parents would initiate, advance, and complete the education of their children in a socially and morally appropriate manner, there would be no need for schools to become involved in this subject. The fact, though, is that all too many parents are either unable or unwilling to dedicate themselves sufficiently to the education of their children. Indeed, throughout modern times, schools have supplemented parental education, and stepped in where parents were not available or their contributions to character education were inadequate. Public education for intimacy is no different.

The fact, however, that some of the responsibility for sex education is delegated to schools, does not mean that parents have lost their right and duty to be involved in decision-making concerning the education to which their children are subjected, especially with highly charged and normatively loaded issues. True, parents are not the only ones who have a say when it comes to education; the state, for instance, mandates both attendance and numerous subjects and other matters of education policy. The parents, though, should not be excluded both as a matter of right and because their involvement can greatly enhance the education provided in school.

Parents have a right to be informed and consulted about all school programs. Schools should actively reach out to the parents and keep them informed about their approach to teaching sex education and what issues they will discuss. The parents' right is accompanied by a responsibility of the parents to inform themselves on the issues at hand before they act to curtail a program or urge the adoption of another or seek to remove their children from a given course.

> *If parents would initiate, advance, and complete the education of their children, . . . there would be no need for schools to become involved in the subject.*

Parents should have the right—and be afforded the opportunity—to opt children out of classes on intimacy, but not to block the whole program. This opting-out system requires notifying parents ahead of time about the material that is going to be covered in such classes, the methodology to be used, and other relevant matters. Children who are being opted out by their parents should be given some other assignments in the same period.

At the same time, an opt-in system, according to which a child would only be enrolled in a course if his or her parents provided prior written approval, is not called for. Children should not be denied education of any kind just because their parents are not available or are indifferent to the point that they neglect to act. They should be given full opportunity to act on their values, but not to block education by inaction.

There is an exception to the above policy: The community may take the position that withholding certain kinds of information directly endangers lives. Similar to vaccines, the common good may take priority over parental objections under certain limited conditions. If schools have evidence that in their jurisdiction a significant number of children die from AIDS, and they believe that there is no other way to prevent the spread of the disease among their students, they may require "inoculation" of youngsters against such dangers by sharing with them proper information and devices. This should be done only after the community discusses these matters with its elected bodies and following open hearings.

Schools are but one factor in the societal matrix that affects children's attitudes toward sex. The media, families, adult role models, socioeconomic forces, and numerous other factors affect young people. Educators should make it clear that they cannot single-handedly deliver all the desired outcomes. Educators need to act as agents who endeavor to activate other social agents, calling on them to discharge their responsibilities in this area, become partners of and with educators. For instance, educators should support efforts to improve the messages to which children are exposed on television. At the same time these "other" forces should not be used as a rationale for families or educators to not do their part.

4

Sex Education Has Reduced Teen Pregnancy

Jane Mauldon and Kristin Luker

Jane Mauldon is an assistant professor at the Graduate School of Public Policy at the University of California, Berkeley. Kristin Luker is a professor of sociology and law at the University of California, Berkeley, and the author of Dubious Conceptions: The Politics of Teenage Pregnancy.

Although more teenagers are sexually active than in the past, more are practicing some form of birth control, which has led to a decline in the teen pregnancy rate. No evidence exists that teaching teenagers about sex education and contraceptives leads to an increase in teen sexual activity. If teenagers receive sex education while they are still virgins, they are more likely to delay their first sexual experience and to use contraception when they do become sexually active.

The drumbeat of criticism that eventually drove Joycelyn Elders out of office as Surgeon General in 1994 may be only a fading memory, but the controversies over sex education and contraception that dogged her tenure linger on. To conservatives, nothing symbolizes the illusions of liberalism better than the failure of permissive sexual policies. In the years since contraceptives became widely available and schools began offering sex education, haven't kids become more promiscuous? Aren't births to unmarried teenage mothers soaring? Therefore, conservatives say, the government ought to practice some abstinence of its own and stop sex education in our schools and programs that promote contraception.

But, like so many conservative arguments that appeal to a general sense of social decline, this one ignores some well-established facts. More teenagers use contraception, they use it sooner after starting sex, and they are becoming more sophisticated about its use. Pregnancy rates among sexually active teenagers have dropped, decreasing by 20 percent between 1970 and 1990. Recent evidence also suggests that sex and AIDS education programs in the public schools have encouraged youth to delay sex, limit the number of partners, and use condoms.

Reprinted, with permission, from Jane Mauldon and Kristin Luker, "Does Liberalism Cause Sex?" *The American Prospect*, vol. 24, Winter 1996. Copyright 1996 The American Prospect, PO Box 383080, Cambridge, MA 02138. All rights reserved.

But, conservatives say, increased access to contraceptives and sex education has stimulated more sexual activity among teenagers. These fears were cogently voiced in 1978 by Archbishop (now Cardinal) Bernardin, who doubted, he said, whether "more and better contraceptive information and services will make major inroads in the number of teenage pregnancies—it will motivate them to precocious sexual activity but by no means to the practice of contraception. In which case the solution will merely have made the problem worse."

Was the Archbishop right? For if he was, Americans might have reason to shut down the great enterprise of sexual enlightenment that America launched thirty years ago.

An American transformation

Turning the clock back on policies toward contraception and sex education would return us to a radically different age. Until 30 years ago, it was the policy of the U.S. government to keep contraceptives out of the hands of the poor, the unmarried, and the young. Even information about contraceptives was hard to obtain because of the legacy of the Comstock Act of 1873, which defined contraceptives as "obscene." As late as 1964 contraception was nominally illegal in some states even for married people. Public contraceptive programs, condoms in plain view in grocery stores, and magazine advertisements for contraceptive products were unimaginable. Sex education for many students before the 1960s consisted of a brief lecture about menstrual hygiene (delivered to girls by the school nurse) or nocturnal emissions (delivered to boys by the coach). Where condoms were legal, they were typically available only behind the counter in pharmacies, which often refused to sell them to customers the pharmacist knew or suspected weren't married. Doctors and clinics also often turned the young away unless they could show proof of parental consent.

The pregnancy rate rose because more teenagers were sexually active, not because more sexually active teens were becoming pregnant.

Then, in a remarkably short time, the Supreme Court made contraception legal, and the president and Congress helped to make it accessible. In 1964 the Court ruled in *Griswold v. Connecticut* that states could not ban the use of contraceptives. In the War on Poverty that began the same year, providing contraceptives to poor women became a high priority. Prior to *Griswold*, only women who could afford a private physician had been able to acquire birth control because the Comstock Act had been interpreted as prohibiting, in most circumstances, public expenditures on contraception. Under antipoverty programs, the first recipients of contraceptives were poor married women, but soon teenagers were also included. In 1966 Congress mandated that birth control be offered to any woman over 15 years of age on public assistance, married or not. In 1967 the federal government reserved 6 percent of maternal and child health funds for family planning for poor women, and in 1972 it stipulated that state welfare programs offer contraceptives to "minors who can be considered sexually active." By the mid-1970s, public contraceptive clinics were the first choice of a majority of teenagers and were especially likely to be used by teenagers from poor families and by minority teens. Contraceptives became available through a wide network of public health services, hospitals, clinics, and Planned Parenthood centers—all this, despite the absence of a national health care system.

Although ready access to contraceptives is now part of the fabric of American life, conservatives hold it partly responsible for what they see as deepening moral decline. Among the sources of misperception about the consequences of liberalized contraceptive access is a series of misunderstandings about teenage pregnancy and the use of birth control. Constant references to "an epidemic of teenage pregnancy" suggest that the pregnancy rate for teens is dramatically higher than in the past and different from pregnancy rates among older women. In fact, the overall teenage pregnancy rate rose modestly between the early 1970s and the late 1980s, from 95 to 107 pregnancies annually per 1,000 women aged 15 to 19; it rose a little more rapidly from 1987 to 1991, and then fell in 1992 and 1993 (the last year for which we have data). Changes in the rate for teenagers closely track the somewhat higher pregnancy rates among women aged 20 to 29.

It is natural to assume that a higher teen pregnancy rate means that sexually active young women are more likely to conceive than they used to be, but this assumption is false. For most of the last two decades the pregnancy rate rose because more teenagers were sexually active, not be-

Figure 1: Timeliness of Teenage Contraception

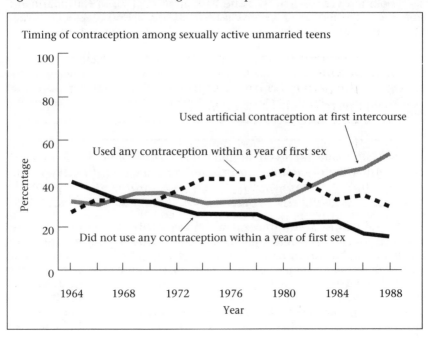

cause more sexually active teens were becoming pregnant. As more teens started to have sex while unmarried, they also became much more likely to use condoms, the pill, and other forms of birth control. "Timeliness of Teenage Contraception" (see Figure 1) tells the story. It divides women who became sexually active as teenagers into three groups: those who used an effective form of contraception at first intercourse; those who used any form of contraception (including withdrawal and rhythm) in the first year after having sex; and those who did not use any kind of birth control methods within a year of starting sex (or, in many cases, ever). In 1964 only one-third of sexually active 15- to 19-year-olds used protection during their first sexual experiences, while 40 percent did nothing to prevent pregnancy for at least a year after their first sexual intercourse. But by 1988, 56 percent of sexually active teens used contraception from the start, and fewer than 16 percent were delaying contraception by more than a year. The unsurprising result is that a smaller fraction of the sexually active teens became pregnant with every year that passed between 1972 and 1990.

Perverse effects?

But what about Archbishop Bernardin's thesis that offering contraception to teenagers increases the odds that they will become sexually active and, more precisely, that they will be sexually active without using contraception? Based on the historical record in the United States and other developed nations, no one has yet been able to show that liberalized contraceptive policies increase teenage sexual activity in general or unprotected sex in particular.

Looking overseas first, we find that almost all European nations report increases similar to ours in sexual activity among teens, although they have followed widely divergent policies on access to birth control. Some have long offered publicly funded birth control to women of all ages as part of their national health care systems. Others make it difficult for even adult women to acquire contraception. These varied national strategies make up a kind of natural experiment. The evidence shows that sexual activity among teenagers is independent of any changes in the public provision of contraceptives.

No one has yet been able to show that liberalized contraceptive policies increase teenage sexual activity in general or unprotected sex in particular.

In the United States the policy changes of the 1960s and 1970s responded to social changes already under way. Young people were delaying marriage but not forgoing sex. In the early 1950s American women had a one-in-two chance of being married by the age of twenty. After 1960 the median age at marriage rose four years, lengthening by about 50 percent the time that sexually mature young women (and men) are single. Norms about sex and marriage changed, and the rate of sex outside of marriage increased accordingly. As "Sex Before Subsidies" shows (see Figure 2), the proportion of American adolescents who were sexually active and unmarried was growing steadily before any public subsidy for birth control. Not only was teen sex already on the increase, but sexual activity leveled off as funding became relatively generous in the 1970s.

Figure 2: Sex Before Subsidies

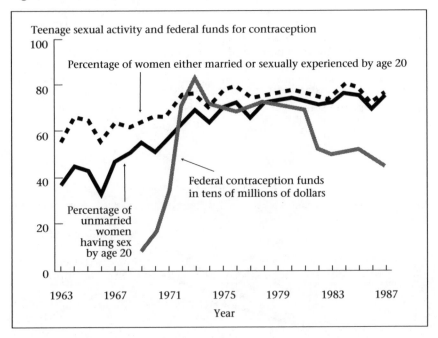

Thus the first part of Archbishop Bernardin's hypothesis—providing contraception increases sexual activity—is unsupported by the available data. His second claim, that as more teens become sexually active more of them engage in unprotected sex, was somewhat true during the 1970s but not during the 1980s (when our data end).

"Unprotected Teen Sex Rises, Then Declines," (see Figure 3) shows the trends between 1964 and 1988 in the sexual behavior of all young women aged 15 to 19. The proportion of all teens who were sexually active and who waited some months to use contraception did indeed grow between 1964 and 1980, but their numbers fell during the 1980s. In contrast, the proportion using contraceptives at first intercourse increased rapidly and continuously over the entire period. And the number of hard-core non-contraceptors—those who were having sex but waited at least a year to use a method—did not increase at all between 1964 and 1980, remaining at around only 5 percent of all teens.

In short, as more young unmarried women have become sexually involved, they have also become more likely to use contraception. And while unmarried virgins are less numerous among teens than they used to be, they still remain in the majority. It is married teens who have almost vanished from the landscape.

These data, however, cut two ways. While public funding of contraception has not caused more teens to have sex, neither is there any clear correlation between public funds and teenage use of contraceptives. When federal funds were cut in the 1980s, overall teenage contraceptive use did not decline too, although these broad national data may not pick up the difference public funding makes in low-income and minority communities. Clearly, other factors affect the use of contraceptives: the determination of many teens to avoid pregnancy; increased commercial access to contraceptives in large anonymous drugstores and supermarkets, and the dissemination of knowledge about birth control—including sex education programs in schools and throughout the community that conservatives have also attacked.

Figure 3: Unprotected Teen Sex Rises, Then Declines

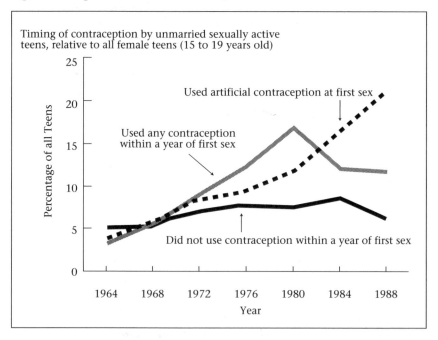

Timing of contraception by unmarried sexually active teens, relative to all female teens (15 to 19 years old)

Used artificial contraception at first sex

Used any contraception within a year of first sex

Did not use contraception within a year of first sex

Percentage of all Teens

Year

Critics claim that sex education has failed primarily on the basis of research that has shown no appreciable difference in behavior between students who have taken sex education courses and those who have not. But only in recent years have most schools offered education about birth control to young teens, timed to occur before most of them are sexually active.

For many young people, sex education has come from a partner, not from a class. In the 1988 National Survey of Family Growth—the most recent, large-scale survey available—almost half of all young women (44 percent) born between 1963 and 1965 had sex education about contraception after they had become sexually active. But as schools became willing to teach sex education in lower grades, this pattern began to change. Of teens born between 1966 and 1968, 38 percent had sex before sex education, but of those born between 1971 and 1972, only 19 percent had been sexually active prior to any instruction about contraception.

Most types of sex education offered after sexual initiation have little effect on behavior. Yet the popular view that sex education does not work was based on early studies that did not distinguish youngsters who received sex education from those who sat through the instruction when they were already having sex. Any beneficial effects of sex education on the students who were still virgins were likely masked by the absence of effects among the sexually active.

Our own analyses of the 1988 survey data show a strong relationship between prior sex education and contraceptive use by teens. We found a difference of about 10 percentage points in the likelihood of contraceptive use. By 1988 young women who had had sex education were only half as likely as those who had not to delay contraception for a year or more.

Young women who had had sex education were only half as likely as those who had not to delay contraception for a year or more.

The impact of sex education stems from small changes among many students. It can hasten their use of birth control, encourage more effective methods, and (though this is not our theme here) help students to resist premature or unwanted sexual activities. In short, it will nudge some students—not all—in the direction of safer behavior.

Some, of course, do not need to be nudged in school. Half of sexually active teens in the 1980s used some type of contraception at first sex even without formal sex education. Others cannot be reached even through a good program. About 3 percent of students who had had sex education had never used contraceptives even though they had been sexually active for more than a year. But between these extremes lie half of sexually active youth, whose behavior can be shaped by the information, skills, peer expectations, and adult counsel that constitute an effective sex education curriculum.

Designing sex education programs

While these graphs suggest that sex education can work, aggregate data tell us nothing about what goes into an effective program. Fortunately, thanks to a panel of 14 national experts convened at the request of the Centers for Disease Control (CDC) and a recent analysis for the Office of Technology Assessment (OTA), we know more than ever before on this question. Under the leadership of Douglas Kirby of ETR Associates, the panel carefully reviewed the evaluations of 16 school-based programs and 7 studies using national data with an eye to establishing what works. Kirby subsequently reviewed an additional 33 studies for the OTA.

Both reviews first address the Bernardin hypothesis that sex education increases sexual activity among teens. None of the evaluated curricula hastened sexual intercourse or increased its frequency among participating students. Kirby and colleagues are unequivocal: "These data strongly support the conclusion that sexuality and AIDS education curriculums that include discussions of contraception in combination with other topics—such as resistance [to sexual pressure] skills—do not hasten the onset of intercourse." In fact, even those sex education programs associated with school-based clinics, which provide birth control to students, did not find that rates of sexual initiation went up.

Indeed, the news is that sometimes sex education can postpone sexual initiation if the program is based on carefully evaluated strategies and is offered to groups of students who are mostly still virgins. Kirby and colleagues note that "two curriculums that specified delaying the onset of intercourse as a clear goal . . . successfully reduced the proportion of sexually inexperienced students who initiated sex during the following 12 to 18 months. Notably, both groups also received instruction on contraception." This result may not have been found in earlier research into sex education because until recently, most curricula did not explicitly seek to discourage students from initiating sex at young ages.

Other programs that successfully influenced student behavior were focused on increasing contraceptive use or, more specifically, increasing condom use, among participating students. These programs had several features in common. They had clear goals and a relatively narrow focus, whether on postponing sexual involvement or on reducing risks of pregnancy or sexually transmitted diseases. They acknowledged the importance of peer group behavior in student learning. They offered accurate information through experiential exercises designed to let students personalize the information. And they let students practice skills in sexual communication, negotiation, and refusal.

In part because of their controversial character, the early sex education curricula that addressed contraception were often forced to adopt a tone of value neutrality, focusing on clinical information to the exclusion of the social, emotional, and moral aspects of sex. The research by Kirby and his colleagues suggests that this strategy was a mistake. In many respects, the most successful sex education programs are liberal in the breadth of their discussion but conservative in their directive message.

Sex education can postpone sexual initiation if the program is based on carefully evaluated strategies.

The Europeans reached this conclusion first. They have carved out a middle ground between absolute prohibition of adolescent sexuality and the total abdication of any adult responsibilities for guiding it. The new sex education programs in the United States are trying to create an analogous middle ground. Feminists and conservatives alike can find something to admire in programs that encourage young women (and men) to resist peer pressure and take responsibility when and if they feel truly ready for sexual intimacy. While the far right will still insist on a policy of "just say no" and sexual libertarians will resent any attempt to tell adolescents what to do, the emerging consensus of the middle has much to recommend it.

The CDC's team of reviewers emphasizes that we are just beginning to understand which factors contribute most to the overall success of the programs. Their main message is that some programs do work and that the next generation of programs should take advantage of the lessons that varied approaches teach.

Changing needs

American youngsters in the 1990s face a different world from the one that confronted their parents. More young people are sexually active, and more report that some sexual activity is coerced. Sexually transmitted diseases that threaten health and fertility (gonorrhea and chlamydia) or life itself (AIDS) afflict many young as well as older people. Helping teens handle these challenges isn't easy. Their needs change rapidly as they mature: A youngster may need encouragement to postpone sexual involvement when she or he is fifteen, easy access to contraceptives when he or she is eighteen, and, throughout, increasingly sophisticated help in sexual negotiation and refusal.

It is simplistic, and mistaken, to claim that the efforts of the past two decades to help teens [prevent pregnancy] have been either ineffective or counterproductive.

America has a long way to go before our teenagers are as effective in preventing pregnancy as are most of their European counterparts. While we understand the desire of many people to turn the clock back to a simpler age, the crucial task now is to continue studying open-mindedly what works for adolescents, and for whom it works. It is simplistic, and mistaken, to claim that the efforts of the past two decades to help teens have been either ineffective or counterproductive. Young people from across the social spectrum have taken advantage of public policies to help them take care of themselves. Legally imposed barriers that once imperiled their well-being have been lowered or removed. That these new policies and programs have made only slow and partial progress is evidence for strengthening them and designing them more intelligently. To abandon the effort now would be a kind of collective, parental irresponsibility.

5

Sex Education Programs Are Ineffective at Reducing Teen Pregnancy

James Likoudis

James Likoudis is a freelance writer.

School sex-education programs that emphasize contraception and values-free information have failed to reduce pregnancy or promiscuity in both teenagers and adults. The traditional values of chastity and abstinence have been sacrificed for the new attitudes of sexual permissiveness inherent in these sex-education programs. These destructive sex-education materials should be removed from the schools and the values of abstinence and chastity taught instead.

Simply put, school sex education has not worked. The statistics are in, and have been for some time, to the alarm of those parents who discover that they have been deceived by the relentless propaganda for sex education that developed in the late 1960s. For 30 years, they were promised that classroom sex education was the answer to a sexual revolution which threatened the morals of their children. The facts of moral and sociocultural decay have been neatly collected in William J. Bennett's *The Index of Leading Cultural Indicators: Facts and Figures on the State of American Society*.

Clearly, formal classroom sex education has failed dismally to decrease sexual promiscuity and sexual deviance among either adults or youths. The startling increases in teenage pregnancies, illegitimate births, divorce, contraceptive usage, abortion, rape, child molestation, prostitution, and more than 20 new sexually transmitted diseases (including the dreaded AIDS) have all given the lie to the various myths that sex educators and sexologists have propagated: 1) that ignorance was the cause of teenage pregnancies; 2) that a neutral, values-free sex education would result in an enhanced sense of personal responsibility in those provided with contraceptive "information"; and 3) that the moral relativism en-

Reprinted from James Likoudis, "End the Mythology of Sex Education," *The Wanderer*, December 12, 1996, by permission of *The Wanderer*.

shrined in formal sex education school curricula would not lead to more sexual license and its ill consequences—broken lives, broken homes, marriages, and families.

Those courageous educators who held fast to those traditional values which acknowledged that there was a religious and moral dimension to any education in human sexuality also understood that school sex instruction indoctrinating students in attitudes of sexual permissiveness involved a horrendous invasion of a child's right to privacy as well as of the parents' right to be the teachers of their own children in this extremely important and delicate area of personal conviction. Schools which introduced and gloried in clinical and offensive Swedish-style sex education curricula with their "scientific" pretensions were rightly seen to verge dangerously on pornography (given their questionable focus on sexual biology and genital behavior in addition to tampering with the emotional affectivity of the young).

Clearly, formal classroom sex education has failed dismally to decrease sexual promiscuity and sexual deviance among either adults or youths.

The beautiful and noble virtue of chastity has not been served well by public school sex education programs which blatantly distort the very meaning of sex as understood in the Judeo-Christian tradition. But it is not only in the area of sex education that public school education has been a glaring failure. Drug, alcohol, and tobacco education in schools have been similar disasters. U.S. government studies reveal the increased crime, violence, vandalism, gang warfare, drug-pushing, drunkenness, cigarette smoking, and allegations of sexual abuse disgracing the nation's public schools.

The Vatican's new document

The entire mythology giving rise to modern sex education has now been exploded by the Vatican's new document, *The Truth and Meaning of Human Sexuality*, released in December, 1995. Articles appearing in the nation's press have not done justice to the importance and scope of this impressive document issued by the Pontifical Council for the Family. Therein the Catholic Church directly challenges the false assumptions and premises underlying modern sex education, but also gives a clarion call to all parents to oppose and to remove destructive sex education programs that are designed to "liberate" young people from the objective moral order designed by God for marriage and family life.

The Church makes it clear that she cannot accept a basically secular humanist sex education that features a clinical and mechanical sexology and a curriculum approach to which parents are made slavishly subject. Parents have the moral right to supervise and control the sexual education of their children, and they also have the obligation to safeguard their children from any explicit, graphic, erotic, and provocative material that may disturb them spiritually and emotionally.

While "sex education"—in the sense of the cultivation in students of growth toward chaste manhood and womanhood through instruction in the moral teachings of the Church—remains, as always, a function of the Catholic schools, the new document excludes any classroom sex instruction that presents intimate sexual details of genital behavior apt to raise erotic images in the minds of young students. It also censures the nauseating "safe sex" and condom distribution programs that undermine parental rights and directly offend the modesty and chastity of students.

It has been disturbing, however, to witness how the intent, scope, and significance of the new Vatican document have suffered distortion in some sectors of the Catholic press.

As an invited participant in the Pontifical Council for the Family's International Meeting of Experts on Sex Education (held in Rome in January 1995 to discuss the import of its new document), I was witness to the consensus affirming that both the spirit and the letter of the Vatican document clearly prohibit the classroom sex education programs that have been in vogue in public and Catholic schools the last three decades. In fact, the Pontifical Council for the Family encourages all parents to exercise their primary rights in sex education by calling for the removal of objectionable programs of sex education from any school which would dare to impose explicit and graphic texts and materials upon youngsters.

Once again, the Catholic Church challenges all educators to safeguard and defend the rights of the family in the matter of sexual education and not to usurp those rights. In this new document, the Catholic Church has once again come to the defense of the family, this time against the kind of demagoguery that has made much of modern education a spiritual wasteland.

6

Sex Education Promotes Teen Pregnancy

Jacqueline R. Kasun

Jacqueline R. Kasun is a professor of economics at Humboldt State University in Arcata, California, and the author of The War Against Population.

Premarital sexual activity, teen pregnancies, and sexually transmitted diseases have risen with the increase in explicit sex-education programs in the schools. Thus, little evidence exists that sex education reduces teen sex and illegitimacy as its supporters claim. The best way to reduce teen sex, pregnancy, and abortion rates is to restrict government-funded birth control and abortions.

During the debate over her confirmation in 1993, Surgeon General Joycelyn Elders sketched her strategy for combating teen pregnancies and sexually transmitted diseases with her usual sledgehammer bluntness: "I tell every girl that when she goes out on a date—put a condom in her purse." Dr. Elders lamented that schools teach youngsters how to drive but "don't tell them what to do in the back seat."

In fact, they do, and have been doing so for decades in the form of explicit sex-education programs and school-based clinics. And that is the problem. Premarital sexual activity and pregnancy have increased in step with the increase in the programs. One of every 10 teenage girls in the United States now becomes pregnant each year. Studies published by the government family planners indicate that these problems are very likely the result of their programs. For example, one such study found that contraceptive education increased the odds of 14-year-olds starting intercourse by 50 percent.

Sex education for all

None of these facts has ruffled Dr. Elders and her allies in the Clinton Administration. Dr. Elders has called for greatly expanding the government commitment to comprehensive sex education from kindergarten through

Reprinted from Jacqueline R. Kasun, "Condom Nation: Government Sex Education Promotes Teen Pregnancy," *Policy Review*, Spring 1994, by permission of *Policy Review*, a publication of The Heritage Foundation.

12th grade, though the surgeon general prefers starting at age three. She wants free contraceptives and abortion referrals through schools and clinics. In his first weeks of office, President Clinton extended the services of federal family-planning clinics and increased their budgets by $100 million. His proposal for health-care reform gives a prominent place to school clinics.

The Clinton administration's expansion of family planning is only the most recent step in a long march of government-engineered sex education. In 1964 a private coalition of educators and activists founded the Sex Information and Education Council of the United States (SIECUS) to "expand the scope of sex education to all age levels and groups." Since then, its curriculum has helped form the basis for sex-ed guidelines in most public schools. In 1965 Congress began to subsidize birth control for the poor. Beginning in 1967, Congress enacted program after program to extend government birth control. This culminated in the Adolescent Pregnancy Act of 1978, which specifically targeted teenagers, even though they were covered in other programs.

Today, sex education is taught from kindergarten through college throughout the nation. In New York, second-graders stand before their classes to name and point to their genital organs. In California, children model genital organs in clay and fit condoms on cucumbers. From such books as *Changing Bodies, Changing Lives,* children are learning alternative forms of sexual expression—including oral sex, anal sex, masturbation, and homosexuality.

At the same time, government-supported "family planning" clinics have blanketed the country, providing young, unmarried men and women with pills, condoms, and abortions—usually without parental notification. School-based clinics, 24 of them in Arkansas alone, often make condoms and other birth-control devices available to children, and even refer teenage girls for abortions without their parents' knowledge. The number of school-based clinics has grown from 12 in 1980 to at least 325 in 1993, according to the Center for Population Options. All told, federal and state expenditures for contraceptive services increased from $350 million in 1980 to $645 million in 1992—not including abortions, sterilizations, and most sex education.

A record of failure

It is bad enough that public money is being used to advance a sexuality agenda that many families find objectionable. What is inexplicable is that these government efforts continue—trumpeted by our nation's chief medical officer—in the face of mounting and irrefutably negative evidence.

Proponents of sex education argue that government family planning increases the use of contraceptives. It does, but it is most effective at encouraging higher rates of sexual activity, teen pregnancies, and sexually transmitted diseases.

As early as 1980, Melvin Zelnik and John F. Kantner reported in the September/October issue of *Family Planning Perspectives,* a publication of the Alan Guttmacher Institute, that the proportion of metropolitan teenage women who had premarital sex rose from 30 percent in 1971 to 50 percent in 1979. They also reported that the premarital pregnancy rate was increasing even faster than premarital sex activity, despite the increasing availability and use of contraceptives. All of this occurred after more than a decade of increasing sex instruction in public schools.

Studies in the 1980s revealed similar trends. A 1986 Louis Harris poll commissioned by Planned Parenthood found that 64 percent of 17-year-olds who had contraceptive instruction had engaged in intercourse; the proportion was 57 percent for those who had not had the instruction. Two massive studies of the effects of sex education, published in *Family Planning Perspectives* in 1986, found that young people who had received sex education were more likely to engage in sex at an early age than those who had not received the instruction. These studies were based on two large national probability samples, giving them a high degree of reliability.

School-based clinics

The record has been equally poor for school-based clinics. Douglas Kirby, a supporter of school clinics, published in the January/February 1991 issue of *Family Planning Perspectives* an evaluation of six clinics that tried to reduce pregnancy by providing birth control services to students. The clinics were operating on school grounds in Dallas, Texas; San Francisco, California; Gary, Indiana; Muskegon, Michigan; Jackson, Mississippi; and Quincy, Florida. Mr. Kirby and his comrades reported that the clinics did not reduce pregnancy. Despite this, they suggested ways to improve the effectiveness of the clinics, which included "more outreach."

As an expert witness, I submitted an affidavit to the Supreme Court of the State of New York in 1991; in it I reviewed seven published studies of the outcomes of programs to reduce pregnancy by providing sex education, together with easy access to contraceptives. The programs had been undertaken in Los Angeles, Baltimore, New York, Cleveland, Seattle, Denver, Atlanta, Pittsburgh, St. Paul, and an unnamed "large midwestern city." None of the seven studies presented valid evidence of reductions in pregnancy: Some gave evidence of increases in pregnancy; six of the seven gave evidence of increases in sexual activity.

Premarital sexual activity and pregnancy have increased in step with the increase in the [sex education] programs.

The Baltimore school clinic program, despite its positive media coverage, needs to be revisited. Laurie Zabin and Janet Hardy, its director, have written several articles and a book about the clinic, claiming it reduced sexual activity and pregnancy among its student clients. However, a careful look at their research methods shows that they manipulated their sample; they omitted the 12th grade from some of their calculations, on the grounds that some of the young women were not sufficiently "motivated" or "advanced"—whatever that means.

Clinic officials have claimed that students "delayed" sexual activity and that teen pregnancies declined. But they based these claims on questionnaires collected from only 96 of the 1,033 girls surveyed at the beginning of the clinic program. They published figures showing that teen sex increased during the operation of the program, but then denied this is what the figures meant.

Last year, Mr. Kirby and others reported on the almost 20 years of experience in the much-publicized St. Paul school clinics, which provide a "full range of reproductive health services," including sex education and prescriptions for birth control. The media have broadcasted claims of significant reductions in student birth rates. Mr. Kirby and his co-authors, however, found "a statistically significant increase in birthrates after the clinics opened." They caution, nevertheless, that the appropriate conclusion is that "the St. Paul clinics had little impact on birthrates." Incredibly, the Center for Population Options concluded that the results prove the need for more "interventions."

Subsidizing illegitimacy and abortion

Such interventions, however, are simply giving us higher rates of casual sex and illegitimacy. The statistical evidence has been around a long time. Susan Roylance studied 15 states with similar social-demographic characteristics and rates of teenage pregnancy in 1970; in testimony to Congress in 1981 she reported that those with the highest expenditures on family planning showed the largest increases in abortions and illegitimate births among teenagers between 1970 and 1979.

In 1992, I conducted a study of welfare dependency in the 50 states based on data for the mid-1980's (the data for such a study become available only after a lag of three to five years). The results showed that states which spent *more* on birth control per woman ages 15 to 44 had higher proportions of births out-of-wedlock and higher rates of teenage pregnancy and welfare dependency two years later.

The study also showed that states which provide government-funded abortions do not achieve lower levels of welfare dependency or a lower proportion of births out of wedlock. Instead, those states have significantly higher rates of teenage pregnancy. In *Family Planning Perspectives* of November/December 1990, Shelly Lundberg and Robert D. Plotnick reported similar evidence that easy access to abortion is associated with higher rates of white teenage pregnancy. They also found that easier access to contraceptives and abortions and more generous public assistance are associated with higher rates of premarital births among white teenagers.

The Clinton administration continues to ignore what can no longer be ignored: Government sex-ed programs and school-based clinics either increase teenage sexual activity, pregnancies, and abortion or—at best— have no significant impact. The surgeon general, of all people, ought to be aware of the ambiguity. Between 1987 and 1991, during Dr. Elders's vigorous condom and clinic promotion as director of Public Health in Arkansas, the teenage-birth rate rose 14 percent.

The Guttmacher Institute, a research affiliate of Planned Parenthood, published an article concluding that "the existing data do not yet constitute consistent, compelling evidence that sex education programs are effective" in reducing teen pregnancies. Reviewing all the published studies on school clinics, investigators at Northwestern University Medical School and the Department of Health and Human Services concluded:

"There is little consistent evidence that school-clinic programs affect pregnancy rates." Even the National Education Association admits that there is "only meager evidence" that sex-ed programs have any effect on teen sex and illegitimacy.

Why, then, the relentless push for such programs at federal and state levels of government?

The near abandonment of common sense and moral instruction of young people in public education is part of the answer. The simple common sense of an earlier era would have suspected that talking to young people endlessly about sex from kindergarten through college, as is now the pedagogical custom, might encourage experimentation. "The philosophy that directs teens to 'be careful' or 'to play it safe with condoms' has not protected them," says Dr. Joe McIlhaney Jr., president of the Medical Institute for Sexual Health. "It has only enticed them into the quagmire of venereal warts, genital cancer and precancer, herpes for life, infertility, and AIDS." Such views, however, are not in vogue among President Clinton's health and education elites.

Another related reason for the adherence to failed sex-ed programs seems to be a stubborn assumption that sexual information automatically serves as a catalyst for transforming behavior.

Government sex-ed programs and school-based clinics either increase teenage sexual activity, pregnancies, and abortion or—at best—have no significant impact.

As social scientist Charles Murray has pointedly noted, however, almost 60 percent of the new white teenage mothers in 1991 were unmarried, compared with 18 percent in 1970. In 1991, 92 percent of births to black teenagers occurred out of wedlock, compared with 63 percent in 1970. Hispanics, who account for almost 30 percent of white teenage births, characteristically have higher fertility than other racial groups. The recent increase in teenage fertility, however, is not the result of Hispanic behavior. Fertility among non-Hispanic white teenagers increased by a third between 1986 and 1991, while the rate for Hispanics actually dropped and the rate for blacks increased only 18 percent. Clearly, the big increase occurred among young—and better educated—white women.

Not only were teenagers having rising proportions of births out-of-wedlock, but as reported by the National Center for Health Statistics, so were women of all ages. In 1960, 5 percent of all new babies were born out of wedlock. In 1991, the number topped 30 percent. This follows nearly three decades of increasingly comprehensive and explicit sex education for our children. Clearly, sexual instruction by itself cannot be expected to promote sexual responsibility. A 1991 *Newsweek* cover story admitted the obvious: "If education alone could affect people's behavior, STDs (sexually transmitted diseases) would be a thing of the past."

What can be done to reduce risky youthful sexual behavior? There is a role for government, but it is largely negative: Restrictions on access to government-funded birth control and abortion have been followed by significant reductions in pregnancy and childbearing. When Ohio and Georgia stopped paying for Medicaid abortions in 1978, not only did abortion decline but so did pregnancy and births among women eligible for Medicaid.

The number of pregnancies among girls under 18 fell by 15 percent within two years after Massachusetts passed a law requiring parental notification regarding minors' abortions. In 1981, Minnesota passed such a law. The abortion rate among girls 15 to 17 years of age fell by 21 percent between 1980 and 1985, the pregnancy rate fell by 15 percent, and the fertility rate by 9 percent. (Planned Parenthood filed suit to have the law declared unconstitutional.) States that have passed parental consent laws for abortion have seen declines in abortion and teenage pregnancies.

Then what explains the flood of claims, so enthusiastically reported in the media that government financing of contraceptives, abortions, and sterilizations prevents teenage pregnancy and saves billions in public assistance? The studies, all disseminated by family-planning interests, rely on assumptions rather than evidence. They presume that if women did not have easy access to subsidized government family planning, they would not restrain their sexual activity, nor would they buy their own condoms, but instead would engage in high levels of "unprotected," sex.

This assumption flies in the face of evidence as well as common sense. Considerable research has shown that people do adjust their behavior to the size of the risks they face. People whose houses are insured are more likely to build on flood plains. Economists have an expression—"moral hazard"—for this well-known human tendency to take greater risks when insurance is more comprehensive and to avoid risk when uninsured. Kristin Luker reported as early as 1977 in *Studies in Family Planning* that women who had ready access to abortion were more likely to risk becoming pregnant.

Government birth control corrupts youth.

In addition, the government ought to end or amend its $800,000 ad campaign on radio and television to get Americans to use condoms. For one thing, the ads suggest that responsible condom use assures a high level of protection against HIV. But the research findings thus far are simply too controversial to make such claims. A recent study at the University of Texas, for example, found that even with condoms, the risk of HIV transmission can be as high as 31 percent.

Some of the ads even serve as an inducement to teenage sex. In one of them, a popular rock star tells the audience that he is naked and that he uses a latex condom "whenever I have sex." Not exactly a warning of the hazards of uncommitted sexual activity.

The second part of a strategy for curbing teen pregnancies is more affirmative. Leighton C. Ku and others reported in the May/June 1992 issue of *Family Planning Perspectives* that young people who had been taught "resistance skills"—how to say no—engaged in significantly less sexual activity and had fewer sex partners than students given birth-control instruction. In an abstinence-based program in Atlanta public schools, students are 15 times less likely to have sex in the year following the program than teens who took traditional sex education or none at all.

Two popular programs, *Sex Respect* and *Teen-Aid,* have done much to slow down teenage sexual activity, according to studies by the Institute for Research and Education. Both teach that abstinence is the healthiest lifestyle and discuss the emotional risks of premarital sex, as well as the risk of disease. A study of Illinois students enrolled in a *Sex Respect* course found that before the program, 60 percent of the students agreed that abstinence was the best way to avoid pregnancy. After the program, 80 percent of the students favored abstinence.

Despite critics of the program, there is a growing market for abstinence-based curricula. A 1990 study of 1,000 sexually active girls under 16 found that when asked what topic they wanted more information on, 84 percent said, "how to say no without hurting the other person's feelings."

Sex-ed corruption

After almost three decades of experience and study, the promoters of government birth control have failed to produce any evidence of its salutary effects. On the contrary, the weight of the evidence, much of it published by its own proponents, shows it to be associated with increases in premarital sex, teenage pregnancy, births out-of-wedlock, welfare dependency and abortion. Most of the young people who are growing up in this era of government family planning are like my students—unwary, basically decent. But there are others. A *New York Times* story in March 1993 featured an interview with a member of a California gang accused of raping hundreds of girls as young as 10 years old. The boy was candid enough: "They pass out condoms, teach sex education, and pregnancy-this and pregnancy-that. But they don't teach us any rules."

The conclusion must be that government birth control is not merely another useless, wasteful public program. If it were, society could afford to ignore it. The conclusion must be, as the common sense of an earlier generation would have predicted, that government birth control corrupts youth.

7

Schools Should Teach About Homosexual Families

Kate Lyman

Kate Lyman is an elementary school teacher in Wisconsin. The names of the children in this viewpoint have been changed.

Homophobia should be treated the same way as racism and sexism—it should not be tolerated in American society. Homophobia and gay and lesbian families should become a part of schools' discrimination and multiculturalism curriculum so that children can learn to be more accepting of those who are different. A photo exhibit of gay and lesbian families in one school successfully introduced the concept that different kinds of families are similar to their own families.

A teacher in my elementary school returned from a conference with information about the photo exhibit *Love Makes a Family: Living in Gay and Lesbian Families.* The colleague had been part of a team of four teachers at the school, including myself, involved the previous spring in the filming of the video *It's Elementary: Talking About Gay Issues in School.*

We were coming together again to make plans to display the photo exhibit at our school. We discussed organizing activities highlighting gay and lesbian inclusion during the two weeks of the display. I fully supported the plan. But at the same time, something inside me balked at the thought of presenting it to the school district administration. I didn't want to relive all the controversy we had encountered the previous spring, when we did the filming for *It's Elementary.*

But a conversation with the lesbian parents of Paul, one of the students in my second/third grade classroom, renewed my energy. We were discussing a protest to be held at a nearby church, which had invited an inflammatory anti-gay minister to speak. They said that they supported the actions of the protesters but that they were too tired to go themselves.

"I've gone to so many marches, so many rallies," said Jane. "There isn't a day in my life when I'm not confronted with homophobia. I'm just tired of it. I'll let the younger people do it for me. More power to them!"

Reprinted from Kate Lyman, "Teaching the Whole Story," *Rethinking Schools,* Winter 1996/1997, by permission of *Rethinking Schools,* 1001 E. Keefe Ave., Milwaukee, WI 53212; 414-964-9646.

I knew I wasn't any younger and was also tired of controversy. But I realized that the photo exhibit was an opportunity for me to assist in some of the struggles they faced every day.

Including gays and lesbians in the curriculum

Although I first became aware of gay and lesbian issues through my involvement with the feminist movement in the 1970s, it wasn't until the 1980s that I began to make the connection between multicultural education, gender equity, and teaching gay and lesbian inclusion. Under our district's Human Relations Program, I had been working for several years on curriculum for Women's History Month, which included not only learning about women in history, but also challenging traditional gender roles. I began to realize that gay and lesbian inclusion should be a major part of this work, and that it also should be contained in the discourse on sexism, racism, and other types of discrimination and stereotyping that fell under the district's multicultural umbrella. "Respecting diversity" were words that frequently occurred in the district's mission statements, a commitment that I was to find out later did not fully extend to differences of sexual preference.

Addressing homophobic name calling, gay and lesbian stereotypes, and heterosexism became even more of a priority when I found myself teaching children with gay or lesbian parents. During the 1995-96 school year my classroom of 22 children was representative of the school's low-income and working-class urban population, with six African-American, four biracial (African-American/European-American), two Asian-American (Hmong), one Mexican-American and nine European-American children. And, as in the last several years, one of my students, Paul, had two lesbian moms.

Although I was continuing with 15 of the students from my first/second grade classroom the year before, this school year had started out tense, with students challenging each other with teasing and name calling. After several days of more minor incidents, this culminated in a fight on the playground. I read a poem with the class (*Coke-Bottle Brown*, by Niki Grimes) and facilitated a discussion about name calling. We talked about the words that had sparked the conflict and discussed how they fell into certain categories, like racism and sexism. Kendra said, "I know a word. It's homophobia." I wrote it on the board and talked about what it meant and how it's related to words that they had mentioned, such as "faggot" and "gay bitch."

There were some negative reactions (among kids new to my class) to the word "gay." Tony said, "I hate gay people." After school he met one of Paul's moms, Anne. Paul went up to Tony and said, "Well, do you like my mom?" He said, "Yeah." Paul said, "Well, my mom's gay, so I guess you don't hate gay people."

Later, I shared with Anne what had happened. She said that she was proud of Paul's efforts to prove Tony wrong. I shared in her wonder at her child's strength and perseverance. Yet I felt uneasy. It shouldn't be up to 7-year-old kids, I thought, to defend themselves and their families against irrational fears and hatred. I felt that I needed to do a more adequate job of shouldering Paul's burden, of helping the students in my classroom to unlearn negative feelings and stereotypes about gay and lesbian people.

From this initial discussion of name calling until the last weeks of the school year, anti-bias education was to become a continuous thread woven throughout our curriculum. The photo exhibit opportunity seemed to be a natural conclusion to our year-long efforts. What was clear to me and to most other teachers, however, as well as to many of our students and parents, was problematic for the district administration. As it turned out, the administration's conflicting messages and muddled tactics, along with full coverage by the local press (our school was in the front page headlines for a week and featured on television news and radio talk shows), succeeded in creating even more of a controversy out of the photo exhibit than I had originally feared.

> *It shouldn't be up to 7-year-old kids . . . to defend themselves and their families against irrational fears and hatred.*

At an initial meeting about the exhibit with the principal, the assistant superintendent, and a parent, we encountered little opposition. The assistant superintendent assured us, "I have no problems with this." However, after consulting with the deputy superintendent and the superintendent, she sent us a letter that implied otherwise. Along with flowery language extolling our "wonderful work" teaching acceptance of diversity and prejudice reduction was this statement: "Having a picture exhibition that highlights all the many different kinds of families would support your SIP (School Improvement Plan) goal, the larger issue of creating an inclusive school, as well as the philosophy of (our) School District. Selecting one family structure only would exclude and not be appropriate given our inclusive goals. . . ." The letter concluded with a suggestion that we meet with interested parents and staff if we intended to proceed with an exhibit within those parameters.

At a hastily called meeting of 17 staff members and seven parents, it was decided that we needed to preserve the integrity of the photo exhibit by keeping it intact. People agreed that mixing in photos of heterosexual families would dilute the message: that gay and lesbian families need to be recognized and celebrated. It was felt that the exhibit would be an opportunity for gays and lesbians to be highlighted, as has traditionally been done with other groups excluded from the mainstream of school curriculum. But despite the decision of this group and letters sent to the administration from the Parent-Teacher Organization (PTO) and local clergy, gay and lesbian groups, university professors, and many parents, the district maintained its stance.

Resistance

A week later, however, the administrators changed tactics and delegated the decision to the school community. They set up a meeting which, according to a local newspaper, *The Capital Times*, they decided was "not one appropriate for (district) higher-ups to attend." The meeting, which was announced on television and in the newspapers as a "public hearing," was called for May 1.

Some of the photos from the exhibit, black-and-white images of racially diverse gay or lesbian families in every imaginable family configuration (extended families, two moms or two dads, single parent families, families with stepparents, etc.), were set up in the school library for parents and other community members to preview. Discussion, however, was limited to two dozen parents who had either volunteered or been recruited by the principal to present different points of view.

The meeting, minimally facilitated by the principal and a district resource person, was described by *The Capital Times* as a "chaotic process." The story began: "A punch was thrown, a moderator lost his cool, and parents were left in an uproar. . . ." Eventually a second meeting had to be scheduled to resolve the issues left unresolved.

Feelings at those meetings were indeed intense. People yelled, cried, interrupted, accused, and sometimes tried to compromise. Having an exhibit of gay and lesbian families was likened by some of the speakers to exhibiting photos of drug dealers or sadomasochists. While many cited religious reasons ("My religion says it's a sin"), a few others gave cultural concerns ("Gays and lesbians are despised in our culture"). One of Paul's moms, Jane, who said later that she was the only gay parent who took part in both meetings, related how difficult it was for her to sit through all the insults and attacks on her family.

At the beginning of the first meeting, our home/school coordinator read a letter signed by 37 staff members supporting the exhibit. The letter said:

Dear (school) community,

If we need to be diverse in our thinking and teaching, then we need to teach and talk about gay and lesbian families. . . . This is not about sexuality. This is about family structure. . . . Additionally, this exhibit addresses a pertinent safety issue. Children are often harassed or intimidated by other children using homophobic terms.

We, as teachers or parents, always challenge a student who is making racist comments or insults. Yet homophobic namecalling—'You're gay!' etc.—is sometimes left unaddressed. . . . If we are to eliminate discrimination, we need to confront it in all forms.

We, the undersigned (school) staff, are strongly supportive of having the *Love Makes a Family* exhibit at our school. We believe it is educationally sound and supports our SIP [School Improvement Plan] goals of prejudice reduction and inclusion.

With the exception of the letter, teachers followed the advice of the union to assert our contractual right of academic freedom by refraining from debate. We joined the observers from the school and the community, who had been instructed by the principal and facilitator to remain silent. About half the parents in the discussion group expressed views similar to those presented by the teachers. They affirmed the need to be inclusive of gay and lesbian families in support of the school's and district's multicultural, anti-bias goals. Several stated that they wanted their children to grow up in a world in which they would be safe from discrimination, regardless of their sexual orientation.

Some parents refuted the parallels to the African-American civil rights movement that had been brought up in the teachers' letter, but other African-American parents supported the comparison. Kendra's mother, for one, said that she had encountered discrimination many times in her life and knew it well. "I can feel it now, again, in this room," she said in an impassioned statement which received resounding applause.

Several alternative proposals were raised: They included leaving out the words Gay and Lesbian in the title of the exhibit, mixing in photos of heterosexual families, and moving the exhibit to the Reach room (a small classroom out of the main stream of traffic). Gigi Kaeser, the photographer who created the exhibit, and several parents deemed these suggestions unacceptable. "This is another case of forcing gays and lesbians back into the closet," Kaeser said.

Toward the end of the second meeting, it appeared that little progress had been made. The 20 parent representatives had not succeeded in narrowing the gap between their widely divergent viewpoints. Suddenly, however, during the last 15 minutes, they reached a consensus. The compromise was very similar to the teachers' original proposal: to display the photo exhibit in the school library; to provide alternatives to children whose parents requested them; and to communicate with parents. This compromise appeared to be more the result of time pressure, exhaustion, and resignation than of genuine conflict resolution. The meeting was adjourned, but the tension continued—in the stuffy and crowded library, in the halls, in the parking lot, and on the sidewalks surrounding the school.

Reactions from the students

Meanwhile, the students in my classroom were trying to make sense of the conflict. Some children were aware of their parents' support for the exhibit; many of their parents had spoken out publicly. Cassie's dad expressed his opinions in the local newspaper: "Why don't they (the school administration) just say they don't want this in here because it is about gay people?" Jodi's dad was featured in the press as well, because he'd been involved in a scuffle with members of the "Christian Right" who were demonstrating outside the school during the first meeting. Paul's moms lent us their rainbow flag, which we displayed until the end of the school year.

Emily wrote a letter to the local newspaper, which was published.

Dear Mr. and Ms. Editor,

Hi. My name is (Emily). I am 9 years old and go to . . . the school that's fighting about gay and lesbian family posters being up in the library.

Lots of teachers and parents think it's a good idea because it shows another kind of family than we usually see. Some school bosses that don't go to (this school) think it's not OK.

There's some kids that live with two moms. I bet they feel pretty bad about this adult fight and I bet they want the posters up too, cuz it's like their families.

Kids don't really know if they are gay or lesbian until they are maybe in high school. I don't think you can tell yet.

What the people are doing when they say 'no' about the photo essay is called total homophobia. I hope kids don't learn to be homophobic by listening to the adults fight about this.

Here's a little something I can add, "Hey, hey, ho, ho, homophobia's got to go!

After Emily read her letter to the class, the dialogue that followed was far more rational and calm than that of the parents.

Anitra: I didn't know your parents were married.

Lena: What posters are up?

(The student teacher explained the contents of the photo exhibit.)

Gay and lesbian families need to be recognized and celebrated.

Cassie: I wanted to stay at the meeting, but my parents wouldn't let me. I think they should go up so people would know that being gay or lesbian isn't bad and then they wouldn't hate them.

Ian: You should fax your letter to all the schools in (our city)!

Samantha: I think two things. I do think they should go up. People can learn that they're not bad, but just the same as us. But I think that there shouldn't only be one kind of family. Just showing them gay and lesbian families looks like they're different and they're different because they're bad.

Emily: If it were Hispanic families or any other kind, they'd say it was okay. They're saying no just because they're gay or lesbian.

Cassie: I know why some people are homophobic. It says that in the Bible that gay and lesbian people are bad.

Samantha: It should have been in our school first. A lot of kids tease about being gay or lesbian. Ellen came and reached over me to get something from her cubby and a kindergarten kid who was walking by our room said, "Oh, they're gay!"

Lena: Those kids probably didn't know what lesbians are. Lesbians are girls who love each other and gay means boys. Gay also means happy.

Ian: Oh, I get it. They're together so they're happy. That's why you call them gay.

Cassie: Rob and Tom (a gay couple who are friends with her family) could come and talk to our class about gay rights.

Only two families had expressed opposition to the exhibit. Joel's mom and dad wrote a letter requesting that their child not participate in the viewing of the exhibit. Ellen's mom and stepdad came into the classroom after school one day, arguing that homosexuality was against their religion and family values. I reiterated the importance of respecting everyone in the school community, regardless of whether we agreed with them or not. They left the room with assurances that their child would not be ostracized for her family's beliefs, and that alternative activities would be available for her.

On the Monday morning following the second parent meeting, we went as a class to view the photo exhibit. After all the discord and tension of the proceeding weeks, the actual event felt almost anti-climactic to me.

I had assigned partners and asked the students to go around the library in pairs to look at the photographs and read the dialogues that went with them. I told them to pick a favorite photo to present to the group and, if they chose, to read parts of the accompanying scripts. Gigi Kaeser, the photographer, joined us for the discussion that followed.

During the discussion, I was somewhat distracted, first by the presence of a parent from another classroom who had been very vehement about his opposing views, and second by the uneasy scrutiny of the principal. But I remember how accepting and matter-of-fact the children's reactions were. Far from seeing something exotic or sinister about the exhibit, the students were interpreting the photos and dialogues as what they were: portraits of families. When we had reconvened in a circle, I let each pair of students show the class the photo of their choice and explain why they had picked it. A typical response was, "Because it looks like a very loving, happy family."

Many members of the class chose families with a racial and/or structural resemblance to their own families. Kendra, who has had a struggle accepting her dad's second marriage to a white woman, picked a family composed of an African-American mom, her two children and her white partner. "I like how the kids didn't like their new mom at first," she said, "but then they changed their minds because she made such good cheeseburgers!"

Having an exhibit of gay and lesbian families was likened by some of the speakers to exhibiting photos of drug dealers or sadomasochists.

Emily, on the other hand, laughed when she read from the dialogue accompanying her favorite photo, in which a girl said: "Teachers don't teach the whole story about families in their classrooms. Teachers need to say that most families don't have a mom, a dad, a puppy dog, and a boy and a girl." "That's exactly what I have!" Emily exclaimed. "A mom, a dad, a brother and a dog."

Emily also said she liked the girl's story of how she had dealt with her friends' reactions to her lesbian family. In the exhibit text the girl said: "All of my friends have known about it. Anybody important to me has known about it and is cool about it. . . . If you can't accept my mom, you can't accept me."

Lena, who has never seen her birth father, was attracted to a photo of a woman alone with a baby. She wanted to know how she got the baby and why she didn't have any partner, male or female. "That's just like me and my mom," said Samantha, whose mom also has been her only parent since birth.

After about a half hour of discussion, the next scheduled class, a group of kindergartners, came into the library. I invited them to join our class until we finished, and they squeezed into our circle, some sitting on the laps of siblings or neighborhood friends. Interrupted only by the squeaks of the library book racks and the voices of children from other classes checking out books, the two classes listened attentively to the remaining presentations by my students.

After the exhibit

After viewing the photo exhibit, interest was high, so I decided to ask the class to brainstorm related activities. Someone suggested reading a class book we had compiled during the filming of the *It's Elementary* video the previous year, which was full of stories and pictures about gay and lesbian rights. "That's not fair," Tonisha protested. "We should write stories for a new book!" Other ideas included making pink triangle pins and designing posters for the hallway.

Such activities continued on for several weeks. During their free-choice time, kids made buttons, which they proudly offered to teachers. They started out by copying a pin I had brought in which had a rainbow background and the words "Celebrate Diversity," but soon came up with their own variations in designs and slogans. They used colorful markers to make rainbows overlaid with pink and black triangles and peace symbols. Phrases like "Love one another," "It's OK to be gay," and "Homophobia gots to go!" embellished the pins.

Being gay or lesbian isn't bad.

I also read several books about gay or lesbian families to the class. A favorite was a daily "read aloud" called *Living in Secret* by Christine Salat. Since the book had been suggested by a fourth/fifth grade teacher, I had wondered at first if it might be too advanced. The story, about an 11-year-old girl who runs away to live with her lesbian moms, turned out to be very popular. Students were relating on many levels to the story—to the element of suspense, certainly, but also to the family recombinations, loyalties, and friction that were familiar to many of them. "Read another chapter!" came to be the refrain, as our read-aloud time began to cut into recess and free time.

Adam composed a letter to the editor of the local newspaper. "I think gay and lesbian people aren't respected enough," he wrote. "It's not like they aren't allowed to go to the movies, or restaurants, but it's all most like legal disrespect. I don't know why people have disrespect for gay and lesbian people, because they aren't gay or lesbian so why do they care. I have some advice for you homophobic people out there, don't go out of your homes! There could be a gay or lesbian person anywhere."

On the last day of the two-week exhibit, we went as a class to have another look at the photos. Ian was fascinated by a photo of a gay family with a dog. "They have a Corgi, just like I do!" was his comment. Afterward, we had a quiet writing time to reflect on issues related to the exhibit. As usual, the students chose a variety of ways to approach the topic.

I think [people] should not be homophobic, because it makes gays and lesbian people feel sad.

Ian wrote: "I think people should all get along together. I think they should not be homophobic, because it makes gays and lesbian people feel sad. I think our school should have gay and lesbian photos in our school because lots of kids call other kids names and to educate the kids."

Jeremy related the issues of gay and lesbian rights to racist name calling. "One time I got called a nigger and I didn't like it so I went and told the teacher because I don't like being Called that NAME because it is bad," he wrote. "That's why NAME calling is bad to say (even) when you are just playing AROUND."

Emily wrote a science fiction story about alien lesbians who encountered homophobia for the first time when they visited Earth. "When they got to Earth they went to an A&W restaurant and a teenager called them 'faggot.' That was the first time that had ever happened, so they said back: '*@#$%^&*!@#$ %^&*!' which means, 'We are proud to be who we are.'"

When they had finished their stories, the students worked on drawings to go with them. A crowd started to gather around Paul's table. He was drawing a picture of the Capitol building in our city surrounded by little circles that represented the 1,000 people he and his moms had joined for a gay pride march. As he drew he was counting: ". . . 99, 100, 101. . . ."

As I watched the children cheering Paul for trying to represent all the people who supported his moms, I thought about the progress we had made. In our classroom, gays and lesbians had moved a long way from the "other" status that they frequently occupy in school and society. Gay and lesbian families and individuals had become integral parts of our classroom dialogues and stories. Homophobia, a word now known to all, had become as serious a charge as any other form of discrimination.

On one of the last days of school, Adam and Ian came rushing in from recess, flushed and agitated. "One of the fifth-graders is homophobic!" they said indignantly. "He was teasing us and calling us 'gay.'" I assured them that his teacher would want to hear about it, and, without the trepidation usually shown by members of our class when they approach the 4/5 grade teachers, they confidently marched into the classroom down the hall to report the incident.

I thought back to the name calling incidents and discussions at the beginning of the year, and all the stress and conflict surrounding the photo exhibit. Although as a class and as a school we had felt the divisions and pain, we had come through. The rainbow flag that was flying at our classroom door was a daily reminder of our struggle and testimony to our commitment.

8

Schools Should Not Teach About Homosexuality

Ed Vitagliano

Ed Vitagliano is the news editor at the American Family Association (AFA). The AFA believes that television, movies, and other media that normalize and glorify premarital sex have had a deleterious effect on America's morals and values. The organization maintains that companies that sponsor programs that denigrate traditional family values should be boycotted and companies that act responsibly in their programming should be commended and supported.

A video about gays and lesbians being shown in elementary and middle schools across the United States is a thinly veiled attempt by homosexuals to recruit children to the homosexual movement. Teaching children to be open-minded about gays and lesbians undermines the authority of the children's parents who may consider homosexuality to be morally wrong.

The battle in this country between those holding to traditional morality and those espousing hedonism has reached a fever pitch, manifested in no clearer terms than the ideological conflict over homosexuality. But forget about same-sex marriage, employment discrimination or AIDS funding. There may be no area of debate that causes blood pressures to escalate more rapidly than the question of whether public schools should teach children about homosexuality.

Now the homosexual community has thrown down the gauntlet by unveiling a video entitled *It's Elementary: Talking About Gay Issues In School,* and as its title implies, the video is aimed at the educational establishment. The video is produced by Helen Cohen and Debra Chasnoff, the latter an Academy Award-winning documentary producer. In 1992 Chasnoff became the first woman to openly declare her lesbianism at the Oscars.

The producers went into six elementary and middle schools where teachers and principals are already force-feeding children with pro-gay grist. The narrator says the educators allowed the filming "in the hope of inspiring other educators and parents to take the next step in their own school communities to teach children respect for all."

Reprinted from Ed Vitagliano, "Pro-Homosexual Video Targets Schools," *AFA Journal,* June 1997, by permission of the American Family Association.

The video was funded largely by the San Francisco-based Columbia Foundation, as well as People for the American Way, the Gay & Lesbian Alliance Against Defamation, and the California Teacher Association's Gay and Lesbian Caucus. The film also credits the National Endowment for the Arts (NEA) with a hand in helping to fund the project.

It's Elementary has picked up several awards, including the prestigious C.I.N.E. Golden Eagle for the Best Teacher Education Film of 1996. Targeted to state departments of education and local school boards, the video has been screened in at least six states, and California Assemblywoman Sheila J. Kuehl, an open lesbian, said she intends to have it shown in all 50 states.

The narrator's voice calmly introduces the video while the camera pans over a playground full of children playing peacefully together at a public school. "Most adults probably don't see why schools should teach young children about gay people," the voice says. While that is no doubt true, it becomes clear in *It's Elementary* that homosexual activists see why schools should teach about the gay lifestyle.

It is to capture the hearts and minds of the next generation. In fact, in an interview about the video with a Santa Fe newspaper, Chasnoff states candidly, "What's clear in the film is that the younger the kids, the more open they were. . . . If we could start doing this kind of education in kindergarten, first grade, second grade, we'd have a better generation."

Out of the mouths of babes

"Most adults probably don't see . . ." becomes the theme of this documentary, portraying the ignorance and bigotry of adults—including parents—as the fountainhead of homophobia. In contrast, pro-homosexual statements are heard coming from the mouths of children, shown as innocents who have thus far been uncontaminated by the backwater views of adults.

A student in one New York City school thinks even 5- and 6-year-olds should be given books about the homosexual lifestyle. If parents "freak out," it's only because they are "biased." And a second grade boy in Cambridge, Mass., says an adult who is opposed to lesbianism is not very "open-minded," and in fact is downright "prejudiced." This theme supplies the rationale for *It's Elementary:* keep the discussion of homosexuality out of the hands of ignorant parents, and place it in the hands of an enlightened public school system.

Circumventing parents

Celia Klehr, whose child has gone through her school's pro-homosexual program, has nothing but praise for the curriculum. But what if a parent disapproves of homosexuality? The program is still beneficial, Klehr insists.

"At least this way it opens the topic," she says, "so that you can then teach what you believe to your child." But Klehr's reasoning begs the question—should schools be teaching this in the first place? If a parent views homosexuality as wrong, what is the child to do with a contradictory message coming from another respected authority figure—the child's teacher? A wedge has been driven between the child's two worlds: home and school; doubt has been raised in the child's mind about whether or not his/her parents are wrong.

What if a child simply accepts the teacher's pro-gay view without question, and never raises the issue at home? The moral values of some parents have been effectively undermined by an authority figure at school, and homosexual advocates have won the initial skirmish in the war for the hearts and minds of a future generation.

There may be no area of debate that causes blood pressures to escalate more rapidly than the question of whether public schools should teach children about homosexuality.

Ellen Varella, principal of Peabody Elementary School in Cambridge, Mass., decided that her school would host a "photo-text exhibit" entitled, "Love Makes a Family: Living in Lesbian and Gay Families." She said she anticipated no controversy, because the school community was a "very open and embracing and nurturing community."

The decision did result in controversy, however, presumably among the closed-minded, non-nurturing types. When a friend warned her that she could lose her job over the exhibit, Varella was unfazed. "I felt strongly that the children in this community needed to be educated around this topic," she said.

Perhaps one of the most shocking statements in *It's Elementary* came from Thomas Price, principal of Cambridge Friends School in Cambridge, Mass. "I don't think that it's appropriate that values only be taught at home," he said. "There are social values as well, there are community values." And apparently those critical community values include this one: homosexuality is good.

Enlightened white knights of the public schools

The underlying belief of these social architects is that parents cannot be trusted to convey the truth about homosexuality to their children. The intervention of the public schools is necessary. At a faculty meeting at Cambridge Friends School, the teachers are discussing the results of their fourth annual Gay and Lesbian Pride Day. One teacher admits, "I think that we are asking kids to believe that (the homosexual lifestyle) is right. . . . [W]e're educating them, and this is part of what we consider to be a healthy education."

Some go beyond mere recommendation of advocacy. Take for example George Sloan, principal at Luther Burbank Middle School in San Francisco. Sloan said he believed that learning under a pro-homosexual curricula "should be mandatory" for all students.

At the Manhattan Country School in New York City, eighth grade English teacher Carol O'Donnell listens as one student complains that she is confused about the issue of homosexuality, because her family tells her it's wrong.

Another student agrees that kids hear different things from different places. The solution? "[S]chool needs to give us all the facts, so we can decide on our own what to think and what to do."

Some parents might be disturbed to know that their voice has been relegated to the status of being one among many. Yet it is the opinion promulgated in *It's Elementary* that, when conflicting voices sow confusion, the public school system can intervene with the facts so the children can decide for themselves.

But are they given the facts? And are they really deciding for themselves?

"There's no right or wrong answer . . ."

The introduction to the video tries to calm parental fears, by assuring them that the pro-gay curricula in schools will only be presented in "an age-appropriate way." This translates very simply: rather than discussing sexual practices and sexually transmitted diseases, the teachers will frame the issue as a discussion about tolerance and civil rights.

In New York City's Public School 87, fourth-grade teacher Cora Sangree is reminding her students of a previous assignment, when she told them to paint whatever came to mind when she said the word, "Indian." Now, she tells her children, they are to write whatever comes to mind when she says the word "lesbian" and "gay."

One student asks, "So nothing's right or wrong in this either?" "That's right," Sangree replies, "There's no right or wrong answer."

Those words play well to the casual observer of *It's Elementary*. But a more critical examination of the video shows teachers' subtle but powerful manipulation of the children to draw the desired conclusion.

> *The sight of teachers standing before the entire school body in support of homosexuality has a coercive influence upon children that is frightening.*

In Kate Lyman's first/second grade class the students often do "class books," put together by the students themselves. On this day, Lyman shows the class their latest finished project, entitled, *Everybody is Equal: A Book About Gays and Lesbians*. The computer-generated introduction to their book says, in part, "We made this book to tell people to respect gay and lesbian people. . . ." The teacher thus established the parameters of acceptable viewpoints in advance of the project: if you don't think homosexuality is "equal" to heterosexuality, you don't "respect" gay people.

At one school assembly celebrating Gay and Lesbian Pride Day, a teacher stands before the students and tells them he's gay. Another teacher tearfully tells the children how proud she is of what they are doing, and encourages them to change the world with what they've learned.

At the beginning of *It's Elementary*, the narrator explained, "We made this film to explore what does happen when experienced teachers talk about lesbians and gay men with their students." What happens is clear. The sight of teachers standing before the entire school body in support of homosexuality has a coercive influence upon children that is frightening.

Later Sangree, alone with the camera, discusses her observations about the day's teaching session. The children, she says, are getting a lot of "misinformation" about homosexuals—not only from the culture, but also parents. And, she says, apparently to defuse potential protests, the curriculum does not talk about sex. That, she says, would be inappropriate. Instead, the school is merely attempting to eliminate "stereotypes" and promote respect. "[T]alking about people in different communities, and biases and discrimination and how that affects people's lives," Sangree said, "I think is appropriate."

Here, finally, we discover that there is indeed a right and wrong answer after all.

Stacking the deck

If some of the teachers do not explicitly say that people are wrong when they oppose homosexuality, they do so implicitly. The words "gays and lesbians" are circled on the chalkboard in the third-grade class of teacher Daithi Wolfe, at Hawthorne Elementary School in Madison, Wisconsin. Then, as he begins to write down the words that students associate with homosexuality, a curious pattern develops. Any negative words offered by students about homosexuals are placed on the right side of his circle: "Homophobia." "Discrimination." "Name-calling." "Weird." And, of course, "Nazis" and "Hitler."

But on the left side of the board—apparently the side with the "right" words—are "pink triangle," "rainbow necklace," "same (as real people)," and "equal rights." Such blatant manipulation might not work on adults, but it is clearly effective on children.

Kim Coates, an eighth grade health science teacher at Luther Burbank Middle School in San Francisco, invited two homosexuals to address her class. One of the speakers, a lesbian, starts off telling the students that she didn't come to school to recruit kids into the homosexual lifestyle. Instead, she admits that she came to change their minds about gays. While they may have come to school thinking homosexuals are evil, she hoped they would leave thinking that "gay people are just like me."

And she accomplishes her goal. After the class, some of the students are interviewed, and they admit that the two speakers have changed the way they view homosexuality.

Christians are the enemies of homosexuals

When *It's Elementary* is not pointing the finger at bigoted parents in general, it zeroes in on Christians in particular: the Christian view of homosexuality is highlighted as an example of outrageous bigotry. In one sequence of clips from TV talk shows, two apparent Christians present the view of their faith. One says, "God hates fags." The other: "The Bible that I read says homosexuals should be put to death."

Later, a fifth-grade boy observes, "Some Christians believe that if you're gay or lesbian that you'll go to hell, so they want to torture them." This skewed view of Christianity is no accident. Chasnoff has said that the film was made, in part, to counter the "hysteria of the Religious

Right." But not all religious views of homosexuality are ridiculed in the video. What, for example, is the theological position of Thomas Price, principal of Cambridge Friends School? "We really believe that there's God in every person, and those people include homosexuals, too," he says. In a twist that is positively evil, the children at one Gay and Lesbian Pride Day school assembly are led by a platoon of teachers in singing, "This Little Light of Mine."

If there was any doubt remaining, the moral worldview of the pro-homosexual curricula surveyed in *It's Elementary* is clarified by one teacher in Cambridge.

After saying that students must be taught that all lifestyles are equal, she says, "There isn't a right way, there isn't a wrong way; there isn't a good way, there isn't a bad way. The way that it is, is what it is."

Homosexual advocates have realized that their greatest potential for changing America's mind about the gay lifestyle lies in changing the seed for tomorrow's crop. Varella, in fact, said she allowed her school's photo-text exhibit in the hope that it would contribute to "improving our civilization," because children are the "leaders of tomorrow." With efforts like *It's Elementary*, homosexuals are well on their way to deciding what that tomorrow will look like.

What can you do to protect your children?

Contact your local school officials and teachers. Ask whether this video is being used in your school system to teach children that homosexuality is normal.

Ask your local school board to adopt a policy forbidding the showing of the video in your schools.

9

Sex Education Programs Should Emphasize Abstinence

Joe S. McIlhaney Jr.

Joe S. McIlhaney Jr., a gynecologist and expert on sexually transmitted diseases, is the founder and president of the Medical Institute for Sexual Health, an organization that provides information on health and sexuality.

Teens who are sexually active are at serious risk of becoming pregnant and contracting HIV and other sexually transmitted diseases. Sex-education programs that emphasize "safer" sex are ineffective at decreasing the number of sexually active teenagers. Abstinence-only sex-education programs eliminate the risk of teen pregnancy and disease. Many teenagers will choose abstinence and the safety it provides for their health when the risks of sexual activity are emphasized and explained.

Abstinence. What's so controversial? Parents, educators and communities want teenagers to postpone becoming sexually active, preferably until marriage, because the risks of sexual activity in the nineties simply are too high, right? Everyone agrees that teen pregnancy and sexually transmitted diseases, or STDs, including HIV, cause serious problems. But how to prevent these problems and educate our young people—that is controversial.

We have had at least 20 years of an educational message that says, basically, "If you can't say no, act responsibly." Yet these safe/safer/protected sex curricula have been tried and found wanting in terms of preventing the skyrocketing damage to our teens and their long-term physical, emotional, social, spiritual and economic health.

It is time for an honest and open-minded look at a new sexual revolution: abstinence until a committed, lifelong, mutually monogamous relationship. Most people call it marriage.

Are the problems associated with sexual activity really all that bad? You

Reprinted from Joe S. McIlhaney Jr., "Are Abstinence-Only Sex-Education Programs Good for Teenagers? Yes: 'Safe Sex' Education Has Failed. It's Time to Give Kids the Good News About Abstinence," *Insight*, September 29, 1997, by permission of *Insight*. Copyright 1997 News World Communications, Inc. All rights reserved.

might be surprised. The data are startling. Here are just a few sound bites:
- One million teenage girls become pregnant each year.
- One in 10 females between the ages 15 and 19 become pregnant each year.
- Seventy-two percent of the resulting babies are born out of wedlock.
- Three million teenagers acquire an STD each year.
- One in four sexually active teenagers acquires a new STD each year.
- Two-thirds of all people who acquire STDs are under age 25.
- Eight new STD "germs" have been identified since 1980, including HIV
- One-quarter of all new HIV infections are found in people under age 22.
- Of all diseases that are required to be reported in the United States, 87 percent are STDS (1995 data).

Nonmarital teen pregnancy all too often has a devastating impact on teen parents and their children. Indeed, teen pregnancy has received much analysis because of the long-term effects not only to the mother and child, but to the father, to extended families and ultimately to society. *Kids Having Kids*, a 1996 report from the Robin Hood Foundation, reveals that only 30 percent of girls who become pregnant before age 18 will earn a high-school diploma by the age of 30, compared with 76 percent of women who delay child bearing until after age 20. And 80 percent of those young, single, mothers will live below the poverty line, receive welfare and raise children who are at risk for many difficulties as they grow to adulthood.

Adolescent dads also do not progress as far educationally and earn, on average, about $2,000 less annually at age 27 as a direct result of the impact of teen parenthood.

One other concern surrounding teen pregnancy often is overlooked. Studies from the California Department of Health Services found that 77 percent of the babies born to girls in high school were fathered by men older than high-school age. For girls in junior high, the father was, on average, 6.5 years older. These studies highlight the problem that a substantial portion of teenage sexual activity is more a matter of manipulation, coercion or abuse than anything else.

At higher risk for STDs

In addition to pregnancy, adolescents and young adults are in the age group at highest risk for contracting STDs. Why? Here are two reasons. First, teenage reproductive systems are not yet mature. That is why, for instance, the risk of pelvic inflammatory disease, or PID, is as much as 10 times greater for a 15-year-old sexually active female than for a 24-year-old. PID usually is caused by STDs such as gonorrhea or chlamydia, which often have no noticeable symptoms. PID is the most rapidly increasing cause of infertility in the United States today.

The second reason that teens are at higher risk for STDs is behavioral. The two leading factors associated with STD infection are how early in life someone begins to have sex and the number of different sexual partners someone has. The Centers for Disease Control and Prevention, or CDC, has reported that by 12th grade, 18 percent of students already have had four or more sexual partners—that's almost one in five high-school seniors. With each additional sexual partner, the odds of acquiring an STD increase significantly.

We all are aware of the devastating and fatal consequences of HIV and AIDS. But other STDS have serious, even life-threatening, consequences. Some STDs can cause scarring in reproductive organs, causing infertility. Others can cause [complications] in pregnancy or birth, including birth defects. And having one STD can make a person more susceptible to acquiring others, even HIV. Hepatitis B can lead to cirrhosis of the liver or liver cancer. And human papilloma virus, or HPV, the cause of genital warts, has been linked to cancers of the cervix, penis, anus and vulva. In fact, more women die of cervical cancer (nearly 5,000 annually) than die of AIDS-related diseases. More than 90 percent of all cervical cancer is caused by HPV.

The best that "safer sex" approaches can offer is some risk reduction. Abstinence, on the other hand, offers risk elimination.

One additional fact: Condoms provide virtually no protection from HPV, even when used correctly. That's right! Condoms do not protect against HPV because this virus is passed via skin-to-skin contact and (have you noticed?) condoms do not cover everything.

The statistics for disease and pregnancy are not in dispute. The concern is in what we should do about preventing these problems from occurring and devastating young lives. This is where the controversy starts.

The prevailing opinion for the last two or three decades has been that kids will do it anyway, so we have to give them condoms and contraceptives so they can be protected." Education programs have given a nod to abstinence as the only 100 percent safe choice outside of marriage but then have gone on to spend much time and emphasis on the "how to's" of "safer" sex. The failure rates of contraception and condoms are not emphasized due to concern that these facts might discourage kids from using them.

The bottom line is that although studies show that "safer sex" approaches do not increase sexual activity among students, none of these programs has dramatically lowered the number of teens who choose to be sexually active, who have to deal with pregnancy or who acquire STDs. Nor have they dramatically increased contraceptive use among those who are sexually active.

Even so, isn't it important to promote the use of condoms in school? Let's look at the facts. In the long run, condoms only work when used every time and used correctly. Also, as pointed out earlier, even when used perfectly they provide little, if any, protection from some STDs.

The highest rates of perfect condom use have been reported in two major studies of couples who knew one partner was infected with HIV. In both of these studies only about 50 percent of the participating couples managed perfect condom use during a two-year period. If this is the best these couples could do, even when they knew they were at risk for a potentially fatal disease, imagine the probability of teens using condoms consistently and correctly over the duration of their premarital years.

Research studies vary widely, due to different methodologies and populations, but in any case the news on consistency of teen condom use is not good. Some studies have found that as few as 5 percent of sexually active teens consistently use condoms, and even the most optimistic have found that only 40 percent do. When given a standard set of instructions to which to refer, no more than 50 percent of adolescents typically report that they use condoms correctly. A CDC study found that only half of sexually active high-school students used a condom the last time they had sex. They also found that 25 percent of sexually active teens used drugs or alcohol at the time of their last sexual experience. This, of course, lessens still further any chance that barrier protection was used correctly, if at all. Critics claim that teaching abstinence is "unrealistic," but it is certainly no more unrealistic than expecting teens to achieve ideal condom usage.

Abstinence eliminates risk

Why should abstinence be emphasized in schools? The best that "safer sex" approaches can offer is some risk reduction. Abstinence, on the other hand, offers risk elimination. When the risks of pregnancy and disease are so great, even with contraception, how can we advocate anything less?

There are a lot of sexual-lifestyle options in our society today, but they are not all equally healthy. Schools should promote what is healthy for students. They should set the standard. When standards are low, students will achieve at mediocre levels. They will achieve at higher levels when standards are set at levels that are realistic, but high.

Some students will continue to be sexually active. We need to deal with them with sensitivity and care. But many other students will choose a healthier lifestyle when encouraged in that direction. If students who are sexually active use condoms, they may gain some risk reduction. But they must not leave the sex-education classroom thinking, "I'm being responsible and safe if I use a condom." The school's message must be unmistakably clear: "There is no responsible sex for unmarried teenagers."

Is teaching abstinence realistic? You bet. Let me highlight just one approach: the young women involved in the Best Friends program, founded in Washington 10 years ago. Beginning in the fifth grade and continuing through high school, girls are provided adult mentors, fun activities and social support for abstaining from sex, drugs and alcohol and finishing their education. The focus is on freedom for the future gained by delaying what might feel good now but damages lives later. A 1995 study found that girls in the Best Friends program had a 1.1 percent pregnancy rate, compared with a 26 percent rate for teen girls in the Washington area.

This is the new sexual revolution. The current risks and later regrets are potentially too profound to offer our young people any less than the opportunity to have the very best choice emphasized, explained and encouraged. To present "protected" sex as an alternative to abstinence is inadequate. Waiting for sexual freedom within marriage isn't an easy goal, but the alternative of broken hearts and broken lives from disease or pregnancy makes this a goal worth establishing. We owe it to our teens to tell the truth, to set the standard and to give them our full support toward a healthy future.

10

Abstinence-Only Programs Reduce Teen Pregnancy

Kristine Napier

Kristine Napier has been involved in abstinence education in Cleveland, Ohio, since the early 1990s. She is the author of The Power of Abstinence.

Sex-education programs that emphasize contraception have failed to lower the teen pregnancy rate. Programs that emphasize abstinence, however, have slashed teenage sex and pregnancy rates. Raising children to refrain from sexual activity is a realistic goal. While parents are the most important influence on a child's decision to be abstinent, several support groups encourage teenage abstinence as well.

L ast year [1996], President Bill Clinton proclaimed May "National Pregnancy Prevention Month." This year, there is a little more substance behind that designation. The National Campaign to Prevent Teen Pregnancy, a nonpartisan, nonprofit initiative supported entirely by private donations, has charged itself with reducing the teen pregnancy rate by one-third by the year 2005. Founded in February 1996, the Campaign has just announced the first of many strategies to tackle the problem.

The Campaign aims to create a national consensus that unwed teen pregnancy is not acceptable. This is good news. Pregnancies among unwed teens place mother and child at high risk medically, socially, and financially. Meanwhile, the social costs of supporting unwed teen mothers continue to rise. So public attempts to restore a stigma against teen pregnancies are long overdue.

Just how the Campaign hopes to accomplish its goal, however, remains unclear. Will it focus on contraceptive education and availability, or will it acknowledge the legitimacy and success of the abstinence approach?

We'd better hope for the latter. Contraceptive education has failed to stem the tide of teen pregnancy. According to the Alan Guttmacher Institute, teen pregnancy rates increased an alarming 23 percent from 1972

Reprinted from Kristine Napier, "Chastity Programs Shatter Sex-Ed Myths," *Policy Review*, May/June 1997, by permission of *Policy Review*, a publication of The Heritage Foundation.

to 1990—the period during which "comprehensive sex education" (read: contraceptive education) began and became widespread. In the meantime, we've created a public-health emergency. Not only are rates of teen pregnancy at a historic high, but a shocking one-third of the 20 million annual cases of sexually transmitted disease (STD) strike junior-high and high-school students, many of whom become sterile for life.

Now consider the programs that teach abstinence. In Washington, D.C., Elayne Bennett's Best Friends program is credited with slashing rates of sexual activity among teens from 71 percent to 3.4 percent in the schools that have introduced it. In one year, teen pregnancy rates also have dropped, from 20 percent to 1.1 percent. Teen Aid, a West Coast abstinence program, cut the number of teen pregnancies in the San Marcos, California, school district from nearly 150 a year to just 20. Perhaps this explains why welfare reformers in Congress last year managed to find $50 million to fund similar initiatives.

Contraceptive education has failed to stem the tide of teen pregnancy.

With the widespread failure of conventional sex ed and the growing success of abstinence education, advocates are poised to smash a paralyzing misconception about teenage sex: Although most parents would like their children to delay sex until marriage, they have been convinced that teenage sexual activity is inevitable and uncontrollable. This may come as a surprise to many, but raising teenagers to be sexually abstinent is a realistic goal. All the best research shows that parents are the single most important influence on whether their teens become sexually active. By some estimates, unfortunately, just 10 to 15 percent of today's youth have discussed sex with their parents, even though more than half of sexually active teens, according to a Roper Starch Survey, wish they could.

We are beginning to see a backlash against the notion that adolescent sex is inevitable. True, welfare directors and social scientists continue to dispute the power of an abstinence-only message. But a burgeoning cadre of school districts is embracing the abstinence approach. What follows is a look at several excellent school-based programs that can help parents persuade teens to abstain. They are all much more successful than government-funded approaches that emphasize contraception.

Parents have a duty to lobby their children's schools to offer character-based, abstinence education. But these resources are meant to augment, not usurp, the parental role. I believe that sex education is primarily a family issue. Unlike contraceptive-based sex education, effective abstinence education depends completely upon parental involvement.

A final word of advice: Parents can do a lot to help their children avoid the tragedy of premature sexuality. The key is to behave with utter consistency. It is self-defeating to tell teenagers to abstain, and then in the next breath advise them to use condoms *if* they choose to become sexually active. It's a dangerous mixed message that fuels risky behavior. "Many of my friends' parents say they don't want their kids to have sex," a teenage girl told the *Cleveland Plain Dealer*, "but if they do, to use birth control. By tacking on that 'if,' parents are telling teens that they don't really expect them to abstain."

Best Friends

Based in Washington, D.C., this program promotes abstinence in inner-city school districts by fostering self-respect and sound decisionmaking. Lack of self-respect often contributes to promiscuity and pregnancy. Without self-respect, according to the program's philosophy, it's hard to say no to anyone or anything. Best Friends is based on the concept that the best kind of friend is one who encourages you to make better decisions about your life. The components of the program include:

Group discussions. Girls meet with adult leaders every three weeks to discuss ways to develop a healthy, sexually abstinent lifestyle (as well as one that excludes drugs and alcohol). In addition to self-respect and decisionmaking, the discussions cover love and dating, friendship, physical fitness, nutrition, AIDS, and STDs. The leaders augment these sessions with videos and reading assignments.

Role-model presentations. Women from the community serve as role models for Best Friends girls, explaining how they have made important decisions in their own lives.

Mentor meetings. For at least 45 minutes a week, each girl meets with a teacher, administrator, or other school faculty member serving as her mentor.

Fitness and dance classes encourage the girls to value their overall health. Cultural events and service projects prompt them to explore their communities and set their sights on the wider world around them.

An evaluation released in early 1996 showed a decrease in both sexual activity and pregnancy rates. By the 10th grade, 71 percent of girls in D.C. who did not go through the Best Friends program were sexually active—compared to just 3.4 percent of Best Friends girls. The pregnancy rate for girls in the program was 1.1 percent compared to 20 percent for girls who did not participate.

"This organization's goals are to produce classy, intelligent, respectful, and productive young women," wrote one eighth-grader from Jefferson Junior High. "All girls should go through a program like this, because Best Friends is all about making positive things happen."

Project Reality

This Chicago-based model offers two programs that promote abstinence for junior-high and high-school students, "Choosing the Best" and "Facing Reality." Choosing the Best is a values-based curriculum that gives teens the information and training they need to discover for themselves that abstinence until marriage is the wisest choice. It accomplishes this through eight lessons designed to:

- Communicate the truth about the physical and emotional consequences of sexual activity;
- Build self-esteem so that teens value themselves and their power to make decisions;
- Teach them to resist pressure;

- Encourage open communication with parents.

Facing Reality teaches more than sexual abstinence; it also promotes abstinence from alcohol and drugs. Research reveals that students who are involved in one of these risky behaviors are generally involved in at least one of the others, so addressing all these behaviors together is key.

Raising teenagers to be sexually abstinent is a realistic goal.

The program includes five lessons on human sexuality, five lessons on substance abuse and how it affects decisions to be sexually active, and five lessons on cultural influences that prompt a teen to be sexually active. The latter subjects demonstrate how movies and television portray sexual activity as desirable and free of consequence, how peers can push teens into activities they really don't want to do, and how teens can resist such peer pressure. Parents receive copies of the teacher's guide.

Both programs have been proven effective in changing teenagers' attitudes towards sex. Psychology researchers from Northwestern University's School of Medicine surveyed more than 1,500 students with an average age of 16 before and after they took part in Facing Reality during the 1993–94 school year. After the program, significantly more students said they believed that sexual urges are controllable, that there are benefits to waiting until marriage to have sex, and that even teens who have already been sexually active can benefit from a decision to stop having sex until marriage.

Northwestern's evaluation of Choosing the Best also found that students changed their attitudes toward abstinence. At-risk students showed the most significant improvement. The evaluation showed that 74 percent of all participants said the program convinced them to say no to sex before marriage; and that 60 percent of kids who were already sexually active before the program were, after the program, willing to say no to sex before marriage.

Teen-Aid, Inc.

Teen-Aid, Inc., based in Spokane, Washington, offers several abstinence curricula for students in grades 5 through 12. "Me, My World, My Future" helps junior-high students understand the consequences of sexual activity. Lessons entitled "Right to Say No" and "Right to Be Free" advocate abstinence in an innovative and highly motivating manner.

The high-school course, "Sexuality, Commitment, and Family," is a values-based program that places human sexuality in the context of commitment, marriage, and family. Students come to understand sexuality as a vital part of identity and feelings of self-worth. They also gain an appreciation of the many benefits of remaining sexually abstinent. At the same time they become fully aware of the many risks of sexual activity.

Both programs emphasize and encourage parental involvement through informational literature for parents, called Parent Grams and Parent/Teen Communicators, that describe the day's lesson and suggest topics for parent-teen discussions.

In the school year before a junior-high school in San Marcos, California, introduced the curriculum, 147 girls became pregnant. Two years after the program was first adopted, the number plummeted to 20. An evaluation of students who completed the program in California, Idaho, Oregon, Mississippi, and Washington reports profound changes in attitudes about teenage sex.

Among the findings: Students were more likely to agree that abstinence was the best way to avoid pregnancy and STDs. They also affirmed that premarital sex was against their values and standards and it was important for them to avoid it. Participating students were more likely to reject the permissive notion that sex is OK if their partner wants it, if they are in love, or if they just use birth control.

Saying no to sex outside of marriage means saying yes to a healthier, happier life and a future with greater opportunity.

Higher-risk students (those who had already engaged in sexual activity) responded well to the program. In fact, evaluations of the program in Washington, Oregon, and Idaho public schools found that although all student groups benefited, nonvirgins benefited the most. This belies the theory that teens, once they become sexually active, always remain so. Indeed, the researchers concluded that being able to influence nonvirgins is immensely valuable from a social policy perspective, because this group is most at risk from all the ill effects of sexual activity.

The Moon Area School District in Moon Township, Pennsylvania, for example, uses the Teen-Aid curriculum. Says school-district administrator Paul Gallagher, "We have selected the instructional materials of Teen-Aid to teach abstinence-based human sexuality to our students. We feel it is our job to support the family as the primary educator and have developed a partnership with the family to teach one message—abstinence—to our students on human sexuality. Teen-Aid helps us do that."

FACTS Project

FACTS Project (Family Accountability Communicating Teen Sexuality) offers separate age-appropriate curricula consisting of 30 to 40 lessons on friendship, sex and sexuality, values, risk-taking behavior, managing peer pressure, setting standards, respect, deferred gratification, setting goals, decisionmaking, and the advantages of choosing abstinence. For example, a session on "refusal skill techniques" teaches teens how to say no with body language and dress as well as with words. Concrete examples and role playing help teens apply skills. The program encourages parental involvement by providing a parents' guide. One parent wrote in an evaluation of the program that "FACTS draws kids and parents closer."

Many students, teachers, and medical professionals like William Toffler, a doctor and associate professor at Oregon Health Science University, attest that the FACTS Project is highly effective at fostering abstinence.

RSVP

The Responsible Social Values Program (RSVP) "provides the students with irrefutable evidence that abstinence is the best possible choice for their future," writes Wayne Farinacci, the associate principal for curriculum at a suburban Cleveland high school, in his evaluation of the program. "This evidence is presented in a logical, factual manner without chastisement or feelings of guilt. RSVP gives our students a message counter to that of popular culture."

Utilizing three separate age-appropriate curricula for students in grades six through eight, RSVP encourages teens to practice abstinence until marriage. The program emphasizes that saying no to sex outside of marriage means saying yes to a healthier, happier life and a future with greater opportunity. Dynamic classroom activities teach students ways to say no to sex and shows them the advantages of saving sex for marriage. RSVP also conveys lessons about the importance of family relationships, respect for others, and self-control.

Other exercises expose the high-risk nature of sex outside of marriage. In one activity, several students are invited to reach into a paper sack of wrapped hard candies and then eat the candy they retrieve. After chewing on the candy for a few minutes, they then throw it back in the bag. Other students are then invited to choose a piece of candy in the bag—an offer that they all refuse with comments such as "gross" and "I don't want something used with all those germs on it." Students soon realize that engaging in premarital sex means transforming themselves into a "leftover" and that they are exposing themselves to great physical danger.

A comprehensive evaluation of RSVP in August 1995 concluded that the program succeeds in influencing teens both to regard abstinence as the best choice and to begin to consider the involvement of their parents in this important topic as helpful instead of harmful.

11

Abstinence-Only
Programs Are Ineffective

Debra W. Haffner

*Debra W. Haffner is the president and chief executive officer of the Sex
Information and Education Council of the United States (SIECUS). She
has trained more than 13,000 professionals in sex education.*

Sex-education programs that emphasize abstinence do not prevent teenagers from becoming sexually active. Comprehensive sex
education programs, which give teens the knowledge and skills
they need to delay sexual intercourse or prevent pregnancy or diseases, are far more effective than fear-based, abstinence-only programs. The new welfare program that requires states to teach
abstinence-only sex-education programs is misguided. Teenagers
need information and access to contraceptives in order to grow
into healthy, responsible adults.

Sexuality Information and Education Council of the United States
(SIECUS) supports abstinence. I repeat, SIECUS supports abstinence. But
SIECUS does not support teaching young people *only* about abstinence.

SIECUS's *Guidelines for Comprehensive Sexuality Education: Kindergarten–12th Grade* state that one of the four primary goals of comprehensive education is "to help young people exercise responsibility regarding
sexual relationships, including addressing abstinence and [how] to resist
pressures to become prematurely involved in sexual relationships."[1]

Abstinence is one of the 36 topics covered in the *Guidelines*, and messages about abstinence are included in age-appropriate sections.

SIECUS does *not* believe in abstinence-only approaches to sexuality
education that have as "their exclusive purpose teaching the social, psychological, and health gains to be realized by abstaining from sexual activity."[2] (This is what the newly funded $50 million federal program will
require grant recipients to teach American youth.)

SIECUS does, however, support programs that are abstinence-based—
such as *Postponing Sexual Involvement* and *Will Power, Won't Power*—that

Reprinted from Debra W. Haffner, "What's Wrong with Abstinence-Only Sexuality Education
Programs?" *SIECUS Report*, April/May 1997, by permission of SIECUS. Copyright 1997 by the Sex
Information and Education Council of the United States.

provide young people with clear messages about abstaining in the context of a broader, more comprehensive program.

Abstinence-only sexuality education is not effective. Proponents of such sexuality education make broad claims that sound exciting. They argue that if you tell young people to abstain from sexual intercourse, they will. These "just say no" programs promise to keep young people from developing "too serious" relationships, from being emotionally hurt, from experimenting with intimacy and sexual behaviors, and, of course, from getting pregnant and from contracting an STD or HIV.

There is no reason to believe that these claims are true. There are *no* published studies in the professional literature indicating that abstinence-only programs will result in young people delaying intercourse. In fact, a recent $5 million abstinence-only initiative in California not only did not increase the number of young people who abstained, but, in one school, actually resulted in more students having sexual intercourse after having participated in the course.[3] Proponents of abstinence-only fear-based programs often recite their own in-house evaluations as proof that these programs are effective. Yet, they have not published their evaluations in peer-reviewed literature and are not willing to make them available for review by outside researchers.

There are no published studies in the professional literature indicating that abstinence-only programs will result in young people delaying intercourse.

Comprehensive sexuality education is, on the other hand, an effective strategy for giving young people the skills to delay their involvement in sexual behaviors. Several reviews of published evaluations of sexuality education, HIV prevention, and teenage pregnancy prevention programs have consistency found that:

- sexuality education does not encourage teens to start having sexual intercourse or to increase their frequency of sexual intercourse.[4]
- programs must take place before young people begin experimenting with sexual behaviors if they are to result in a delay of sexual intercourse.[5]
- teenagers who start having intercourse following a sexuality education program are more likely to use contraceptives than those who have not participated in a program.[6]
- HIV programs that use cognitive and behavioral skills training with adolescents demonstrate "consistently positive" results.[7]

Indeed, a recent World Health Organization review of 35 studies found that the programs most effective in changing young people's behavior are those that address abstinence, contraception, *and* STD prevention.[8] In addition, the National Institutes of Health's Consensus Panel on AIDS said in February 1997 that the abstinence-only approach to sexuality education "places policy in direct conflict with science and ignores overwhelming evidence that other programs [are] effective."[9]

Fear-based, abstinence-only programs also fail to address many of the antecedents of early first intercourse. Extensive research conducted during the past two decades has clearly delineated a portrait of a young person who begins intercourse prior to age 14.

Education programs cannot influence some of the factors such as early physical development, lower age of menarche or a higher testosterone level, older siblings, single-parent household environments, or mothers with lower educational attainment.

Sexuality education programs can, however, potentially address other factors such as young people's perception of their friends' and siblings' sexual behaviors, the timing of first dating, steady relationships, and beliefs about gender role stereotypes.

Other venues such as counseling and mentoring programs can address these other antecedents of early first intercourse: lower school performance, lower reading and writing skills, lack of parental support, lower church attendance, depression, and other problem behaviors, such as substance use (including alcohol and nicotine), and school delinquency.[10]

Federal requirement #1

The new welfare reform program requires that sexuality education classes in the United States teach that "abstinence from sexual activity outside marriage is the expected standard for all school-age children." Although adults may very well want this as a standard, it is far from accurate in describing the reality of today's teenagers.

Almost all American adolescents engage in some type of sexual behavior. Although most policy debates about sexuality education have focused on sexual intercourse and its negative consequences, young people actually explore their sexuality from a much wider framework that includes dating, relationships, and intimacy.

The welfare reform legislation never even defines "sexual activity." Since the definition includes the word "activity" rather than "intercourse," one must assume that it is broader and includes a prohibition against other activities besides sexual intercourse. This is, however, never stated. For clarification, the Medical Institute for Sexual Health (MISH) defines *abstinence* as "avoiding sexual intercourse as well as any genital contact or genital stimulation."[11] Other fear-based curricula define it as any behaviors beyond hand holding and light kissing.[12]

The reality is that sexual behavior is almost universal among American adolescents. A majority of American teenagers date, over 85 percent have had a boyfriend or girlfriend and have kissed someone romantically, and nearly 80 percent have engaged in deep kissing.[13]

The majority of young people move from kissing to more intimate sexual behaviors during their teenage years. More than 50 percent engage in "petting behaviors." By the age of 14, more than 50 percent of all boys have touched a girl's breasts, and 25 percent have touched a girl's vulva. By the age of 18, more than 75 percent have engaged in heavy petting.[14] From 25 to 50 percent of teens report that they have experienced fellatio and/or cunnilingus.[15] A recent study found that of those teens who are virgins, nearly one third reported that they had engaged in heterosexual masturbation of or by a partner. One tenth of virgins had participated in oral sex, and one percent had participated in anal intercourse.[16]

More than half of American teenagers in schools have had sexual intercourse. The latest data from the Youth Risk Behavior Surveillance System of the U.S. Centers for Disease Control and Prevention found that 54 percent of high school students had sexual intercourse, a rate virtually unchanged since the study began in 1990.[17] By the time they reach the age of 20, 80 percent of boys and 76 percent of girls have had sexual intercourse.[18]

At each stage of adolescence, higher proportions of boys and girls have had sexual intercourse today than 20 years ago. The largest increase occurred between 1971 and 1979. The increase was modest in the 1980s. It appeared to level off in the 1990s.[19] It is important to note, however, that these trends started much earlier than the 1970s. In fact, the modal age for first intercourse was 17 for men and 18 for women in the 1950s and 1960s. It was 16 for men and nearly 17 for women in the 1970s and 1980s. This is a one-year change over a 40-year span.[20]

Federal requirement #2

The new federal program also requires that grantees teach that "abstinence from sexual activity is the only certain way to avoid out-of-wedlock pregnancy, sexually transmitted diseases, and other associated health problems."

On the surface, it is hard to argue with this statement. The SIECUS *Guidelines* themselves state that "abstinence from sexual intercourse is the most effective method of preventing pregnancies and STDs/HIV." Yet, after learning that abstinence is the "only certain way" to avoid pregnancy and STDs/HIV, young people may get the impression that contraception and condoms are not effective. In fact, many of the fear-based approaches to sexuality education discuss methods of contraception only in terms of their failure rates.[21] Indeed, professionals who work directly with adolescents in schools and clinics can attest that adolescent vows of abstinence fail far more than condoms do.

Messages that contraception and condoms are not effective could, unfortunately, reverse the significant strides that American youth have made toward having safer sex during the past two decades. Consider these statistics:

- In 1979, fewer than 50 percent of adolescents used a contraceptive at first intercourse.
- In 1988, more than 65 percent used them.
- By 1990, more than 70 percent used them.[22]

Teenagers who receive contraceptive education in the same year that they become sexually active are 70 to 80 percent more likely to use contraceptive methods (including condoms) and more than twice as likely to use the pill.[23]

It is vitally important that programs encourage young people who engage in intercourse to use contraception and condoms. According to the National Institutes of Health, "although sexual abstinence is a desirable objective, programs must include instruction in safe sex behavior, including condom use."[24]

Federal requirement #3

The new abstinence-only programs must also teach that "a mutually faithful monogamous relationship in the context of marriage is the expected standard of human sexual activity."

This "information" is clearly not true in American culture. The fact is that the vast majority of Americans begin having sexual relationships (including sexual intercourse) as teenagers. Fewer than 7 percent of men and 20 percent of women aged 18 to 59 were virgins when they were married.[25] Only 10 percent of adult men and 22 percent of adult women report that their first sexual experience was with their spouse, many of whom had their first intercourse when they were engaged prior to marriage.[26] Indeed, this "norm" was probably never true: a third of all Pilgrim brides were pregnant when they were married.[27]

There are currently more than 74 million American adults who are classified as single because they have delayed marriage, decided to remain single, are divorced, or have entered into a gay or lesbian partnership. More than three quarters of these men and two thirds of these women have had sex with a partner in the past 12 months.[28] Most of them would take offense at this new "standard of human behavior." Under this new program's definition, schools will teach young people that these adults must remain celibate throughout their lives.

The concept of chastity until marriage may have made more sense a hundred years ago when teenagers reached puberty in their middle teens. For them, marriage and other adult responsibilities closely followed. Today's young people are different: They reach puberty earlier, they have intercourse earlier, and they marry in their middle twenties. In fact, women and men marry several years later today than they did in the 1950s. The current mean age for first marriage is 26.7 years-old for men and 24.5 years-old for women.[29]

Federal requirement #4

The new federal programs must also teach that "sexual activity outside of marriage is likely to have harmful psychological and physical effects."

There is no sound public health data to support this statement. It is certainly true that sexual relations can lead to unplanned pregnancies, STDs, and HIV. It is also true that intimate relationships can be harmful for some people. But the reality is that the majority of people have had sexual relationships prior to marriage with no negative repercussions. For example, one study reports that when premarital sexual intercourse is satisfying, it has a positive effect on relationships for both males and females.[30] The largest study of adult sexual behavior found that more than 90 percent of men and more than 70 percent of women recall that they wanted their first intercourse to happen when it did; only 6.9 percent of men and 21 percent of women had first intercourse on their wedding night.[31]

The National Commission on Adolescent Sexual Health recognizes that adolescent sexuality is a highly charged emotional issue for many adults. It urges, however, that policymakers recognize that sexual development is an essential part of adolescence and that the majority of adolescents engage in sexual behaviors as part of their overall development.

More than 50 national organizations have endorsed the Commission's consensus statement that says "society should encourage adolescents to delay sexual behaviors until they are ready physically, cognitively, and emotionally for mature sexual relationships and their consequences."

82   *At Issue*

These organizations urge, however, that "society must also recognize that a majority of adolescents will become involved in sexual relationships during their teenage years. Adolescents should receive support and education for developing the skills to evaluate their readiness for mature sexual relationships."[32]

The reality is that the majority of American adults believe that young people need to be told more than "just say no." Although 60 percent believe that premarital sexual relations for teenagers is always wrong,[33] more than three-quarters of adults also believe that teenagers need information and access to contraceptive services and STD prevention information.[34] Abstinence-only programs, which include misinformation about sexual behaviors and promote fear and shame, are unlikely to prove effective.

If Congress and the states are serious about helping young people delay sexual behaviors and grow into healthy, responsible adults, they will support a comprehensive approach to sexuality education that has a proven track record in accomplishing these goals.

Notes

1. National Guidelines Task Force, *Guidelines for Comprehensive Sexuality Education, Kindergarten–12th Grade* (New York: Sexuality Information and Education Council of the United States, 1991).

2. *Congressional Record*/U.S. Senate, Sept. 15, 1995, pp. 513647–9.

3. D. Kirby, M. Korpi, R.P. Barth, and H.H. Cagampang, *Evaluation of Education Now and Babies Later (ENABL): Final Report* (Berkeley, CA: University of California, School of Social Welfare, Family Welfare Research Group, 1995).

4. J.J. Frost and J.D. Forrest, "Understanding the Impact of Effective Teenage Pregnancy Prevention Programs," *Family Planning Perspectives,* 27:5 (1995): 188–96.; D. Kirby et al, "School-based Programs to Reduce Sexual Risk Behaviors: A Review of Effectiveness," *Public Health Reports,* 190:3 (1997): 339–60; A. Grunseit and S. Kippax, *Effects of Sex Education on Young People's Sexual Behavior* (Geneva: World Health Organization, 1993).

5. D. Kirby et al, "School-Based Programs," 339–60.

6. A. Grunseit and S. Kippax, *Effects of Sex Education,* 339–60.

7. J.J. Frost and J.D. Forrest, "Understanding Prevention Programs."

8. A. Grunseit and S. Kippax, *Effects of Sex Education.*

9. National Institutes of Health, *Consensus Development Conference Statement,* Feb. 11–13, 1997.

10. K.A. Moore, B.C. Miller, D. Glei, and D.R. Morrison, *Adolescent Sex, Contraception, and Childbearing: A Review of Recent Research,* (Washington, DC: Child Trends, Inc., 1995).

11. *National Guidelines for Sexuality and Character Education* (Texas: Medical Institute for Sexual Health, 1996), p. 7.

12. L. Kantor, "Scared Chaste? Fear-Based Educational Curricula," *SIECUS Report,* 21:2 (1992): 1–15.

13. R. Coles and F. Stokes, *Sex and the American Teenager* (New York: Harper

and Row, 1985) and Roper Starch Worldwide, *Teens Talk About Sex: Adolescent Sexuality in the 90s* (New York: Sexuality Information and Education Council of the United States, 1994).

14. Ibid.

15. S. Newcomer and J. Udry, "Oral Sex in an Adolescent Population," *Archives of Sexual Behavior*, 14 (1985): 41–6.

16. M.A. Schuster, R.M. Bell, D.E. Kanouse, "The Sexual Practices of Adolescent Virgins: Genital Sexual Activities of High School Students Who Have Never Had Vaginal Intercourse," *American Journal of Public Health* (November 1996) 86:11, 1570–76.

17. *Morbidity and Mortality Weekly Report*, Sept. 27, 1996, 45: SS–4; YRBS, 1990.

18. Alan Guttmacher Institute, *Sex and America's Teenagers* (New York: The Alan Guttmacher Institute, 1994).

19. Ibid.

20. E. Laumann et al, *The Social Organization of Sexuality—Sexual Practices in the United States* (Chicago: The University of Chicago Press, 1994).

21. L. Kantor, "Scared Chaste? Fear-Based Educational Curricula."

22. D. Haffner, editor, *Facing Facts: Sexual Health for America's Adolescents* (New York: Sexuality Information and Education Council of the United States, 1994).

23. J. Mauldon and K. Luker, "The Effects of Contraceptive Education on Method Use at First Intercourse," *Family Planning Perspectives*, 28:1 (1996): 19.

24. National Institutes of Health, *Consensus Development Conference Statement*, Feb. 11–13, 1997.

25. E. Laumann et al, *The Social Organization of Sexuality*.

26. Ibid.

27. J. D'Emilio and E. Freedman, *Intimate Matters: A History of Sexuality in America* (New York: Harper and Row, 1988).

28. E. Laumann et al, *The Social Organization of Sexuality*.

29. U.S. Census Bureau, *Marital Status and Living Arrangements*, March 1994.

30. Rodney M. Cate, Edgar Long, Jeffrey J. Angera, and Kristen Draper, "Sexual Intercourse and Relationship Development," *Family Relations*, April 1993, p. 162.

31. E. Laumann et al, *The Social Organization of Sexuality*.

32. D. Haffner, editor, *Facing Facts*.

33. E. Laumann et al, *The Social Organization of Sexuality*.

34. Gallup Poll, "Attitudes Toward Contraceptives," March 1985.

12

Studies to Determine the Effectiveness of Sex-Education and Abstinence-Only Programs Are Inconclusive

Russell W. Gough

Russell W. Gough is a professor of philosophy and ethics at Pepperdine University and the author of Character Is Destiny: The Value of Personal Ethics in Everyday Life.

Both abstinence-only programs and comprehensive sex-education programs cite studies and statistics to support their claims that their programs reduce teen sexual activity and pregnancy. However, insufficient evidence exists to prove that one method of sex education is conclusively superior to the other. Both sides of the debate have also presented misleading or inaccurate research results. It is also important to determine how researchers define "effective." Finally, values play an important role in sex education and cannot be separated from the research.

Clashes over school-based sex-education programs have erupted like volcanoes over the past decade. Each side has cited statistics and made claims to back up its position, and has jockeyed for attention in newspaper articles, op-ed columns, and TV broadcasts.

But which side's program *really works*: sexual-abstinence education, or "comprehensive" sex ed, which teaches the abstinence option as part of a broad-brush treatment of sexual issues, including contraception, abortion, and homosexuality?

The public-health and family problems confronting society today are stark and disturbing: Over 1 million teenage girls a year become pregnant (with 65 percent of the resulting babies born out of wedlock).

Moreover, 3 million teens acquire a sexually transmitted disease each year (which translates into 1 out of every 10 adolescents).

Russell W. Gough, "Does Abstinence Education Work?" This article appeared in the August 1997 issue, and is reprinted with permission from, *The World & I*, a publication of The Washington Times Corporation, copyright ©1997.

While virtually all Americans agree that some form of proactive and preventive educational measures are necessary to address these invidious problems, varied and passionate opinions exist as to precisely what form sex-education curricula should take.

The reason is that this debate often entails deeply diverging and divisive value-based viewpoints on human development, sexual identity, lifestyle, and abortion.

Indeed, the battle cry rhetoric over how to best address the alarming rates of teen pregnancy and sexually transmitted diseases (STDs) crescendoed to an all-time high this past March [1997]. At that time, the federal government announced it would spend $250 million over five years to promote abstinence-only education programs.

The federally mandated initiative is designed to teach young Americans that:

• sex before marriage "is likely to have harmful psychological and physical effects" and

• avoidance of extramarital sex "is the expected standard" of human behavior.

The legislation, initiated by Congress and signed into law by President Clinton, represents the largest effort ever undertaken by the federal government to promote sexual abstinence outside marriage.

A total of $50 million a year will be automatically released beginning October 1, 1997, to states that apply for it and provide a 75 percent match. (That is, states must provide $3 for every $4 from the federal government.) The program is widely expected to spawn numerous abstinence-only courses nationwide.

Culture clash

Critics of the abstinence-only measure quickly sought to drive home one overarching rejoinder: Sufficient scientific evidence does not exist to demonstrate that abstinence-only programs work. Thus, it was argued, allocating such a large sum of money to such dubious educational programs is scientifically unfounded at best and irresponsibly wasteful at worst.

It would be far wiser and empirically sound, the critics said, to invest in "comprehensive" sex-education programs that emphasize "safe sex" or "safer sex" instruction—practical information on birth control (condom use in particular), various sexual options, and the like—and at the same time teach the advantages of abstinence.

Varied and passionate opinions exist as to precisely what form sex-education curricula should take.

Besides, the critics added, in a significant number of cases it is highly unrealistic to expect teenagers to practice abstinence. Many teens will engage in sex no matter how much we encourage them to abstain, so we are better off providing them with the know-how to have sex safely.

On the other side of the issue, supporters of the federal initiative defended its political merit and educational necessity primarily on the basis of one largely unarguable piece of evidence: The conventional "safe sex" education programs of the past two decades have not lowered the rates of teen pregnancy and STDs.

Such programs have failed in large measure, it was argued further, because of their self-defeating premise that "teens are going to do it anyway." As a result, these programs primarily and often exclusively made it their goal to teach teens how to have sex safely (to prevent STDs) and responsibly (to avoid pregnancy) instead of establishing abstinence as a central aim.

The reliable scientific research to date is far too scant and preliminary to offer us any overarchingly confident . . . answers concerning the effectiveness of school-based sex-education programs.

In notable fact, no school-based abstinence-oriented curricula existed prior to the late 1980s. Conventional "safe sex" programs did not emphasize abstinence until after the discovery of the AIDS virus.

Given that the rates of teen pregnancy and STDs have clearly not been reduced, supporters of the legislation said, it is high time to try a different model of sex education—the abstinence-only approach. Besides, to tell teens, "Don't have sex, but here's how to do it safely," sends a mixed message and is tantamount to encouraging sexual activity.

Accordingly, those who espouse the first general rhetorical argument are advocates of what is usually described as the "safe-sex," "safer-sex," or "comprehensive" approach to sex education. And those who espouse the second general rhetorical argument are advocates of what is variously described as the "abstinence-only," "abstinence," "abstinence-based," or "abstinence-oriented" approach to sex education.

Notably, the latter two labels typically suggest that, while some information regarding contraception use is or may be appropriate for certain age levels, abstinence should be the central and guiding ideal of any sex-ed program. (These latter two labels, however, are now often used by "safe sex" or "comprehensive" programs to convey that abstinence instruction is a part of their curricula.)

Scant scientific research

These two arguments on either side of the federal government's $250 million abstinence-only campaign inevitably press us—policymakers, educators, parents, and concerned citizens alike—to ask the following bedrock question: Rhetoric aside, which approach is most supported by the scientific research regarding sex education?

To be sure, this is a critical question that deserves—indeed, requires—a conscientious and decisive response. At present, however, only a conscientious response is available: The reliable scientific research to date is far too scant and preliminary to offer us any overarchingly confident, much less decisive, answers concerning the effectiveness of school-based sex-education programs.

Beyond the few and strikingly insufficient studies that exist, there is only quasiscientific or anecdotal evidence—which, to be sure, is plentiful on both sides of the debate and which does count for something but is not the focus here. The focus is on the "reliable scientific research," by which is meant methodologically rigorous studies. According to Douglas Kirby, a leading researcher in this field, a sound study should:
- evaluate a sufficient number of representative programs;
- use random assignment;
- include a sufficiently large sample size;
- conduct long-term follow-up;
- measure behavior rather than just attitudes or beliefs;
- conduct proper statistical analyses;
- publish both positive and negative results;
- replicate studies of successful programs; and
- use independent evaluators.

In 1994, in the most comprehensive review to date of the relevant research, Kirby and eight colleagues attempted to assess the effectiveness of 23 studies of school-based sex-education programs that had been published in professional, peer-reviewed journals.

Among the studies, the researchers identified 7 that were based on national surveys and 16 that evaluated the impact of specific programs. Of the latter, the researchers identified 13 studies of "safe sex" or "comprehensive" sex-education programs, and, notably, a mere 3 studies involving school-based abstinence-only programs (which should not be surprising, given that such programs have only been in existence since the late 1980s).

Tentative conclusions emerge

In summarizing their assessment of the 23 studies, Kirby and his colleagues importantly concluded, "There are serious limitations in the research on pregnancy prevention programs, and little is known with much certainty." They nonetheless went on to offer the following noteworthy—but largely tentative—observations about the impact of such programs:

- The studies that were reviewed show that programs involving both abstinence and STD, HIV/AIDS, and contraception education "do not increase sexual activity."

- The seven national surveys suggest that sex-education programs "do increase the use of contraceptives and AIDS education programs do increase the use of condoms somewhat. However, the data are not always consistent."

- "To date, the published literature does not provide any good evidence indicating whether programs focusing only upon abstinence either do or do not delay the onset of intercourse or reduce the frequency of intercourse."

- The few programs that delayed the onset of intercourse, increased the use of condoms or other contraceptives, or reduced risky sexual behaviors had six common characteristics:

1. "theoretical grounding in social-learning or social-influence theories";

2. "a narrow focus on reducing specific sexual risk-taking behaviors";
3. "experiential activities to convey the information on the risks of unprotected sex and how to avoid those risks and to personalize that information";
4. "instruction on social influences and pressures";
5. "reinforcement of individual values and group norms against unprotected sex that are age and experience appropriate"; and
6. "activities to increase relevant skills and confidence in those skills."

Making sense of the research

As with most social scientific studies and data, however, a few important words of caution are in order here, for these types of "facts" do not speak for themselves but require a great deal of interpretation, context, and qualification.

First and foremost, as Kirby and his colleagues make quite clear, their "conclusions" at present are tentative and preliminary at best.

"Our ability to reach definitive conclusions," they said, "was limited by the few rigorous studies of individual programs, by methodological limitations of individual studies, and by inconsistent results among some of the findings. Additional research needs to employ more valid and statistically powerful methods."

As such, one could understandably and fairly infer that the existing scientific literature examining the effectiveness of school-based sex-education programs cannot and should not be used as a rhetorical or political trump card, to say the least.

Second, both safe-sex and abstinence-only activists (to the chagrin of researchers) have drawn—and publicized—misleading or inaccurate conclusions from the research Kirby and his colleagues conducted.

For example, a number of abstinence-only advocates have inferred that safe-sex programs promote increased sexual activity among teens, given that the research indicates such programs increase the use of contraceptives. This does not necessarily follow, of course, as Kirby and his colleagues point out: It may be the case that safe-sex programs do not increase sexual activity and at the same time do increase the use of condoms (among those who are already sexually active, that is).

On the other side, those opposed to abstinence-only curricula continue to argue, citing the Kirby study as "proof," that abstinence-only programs "do not work." But the Kirby study clearly does not demonstrate this assertion.

It makes no small difference how researchers . . . define the concept of "effectiveness."

The most significant conclusion Kirby and his associates drew concerning the effectiveness of abstinence-only programs is that, given the paucity and incompleteness of existing scholarly research on such programs (which, in turn, is largely due to the very recent advent of such programs), one cannot presently say with any empirical confidence to what extent they are or are not effective. Scientifically speaking, we simply don't know yet.

Third, and significantly, an inescapable philosophical point that undergirds the scientific issue is this: It makes no small difference how researchers (much less policymakers and political activists) define the concept of "effectiveness."

For example, in their comprehensive study, Kirby and his associates—consistent with "safe sex" or "comprehensive" sex-ed advocates but not with most "abstinence-only" or "abstinence-primarily" advocates—define "effectiveness" quite narrowly (and, I should be quick to add, understandably for empirical purposes) in terms of reducing teen pregnancies and STDs. But many individuals and groups that back abstinence instruction tend to construe "effectiveness" in terms of a broader range of outcomes—not merely the physical-health outcomes of reducing teen pregnancies and STDs but also outcomes related to emotional, psychological, spiritual, and "character" consequences.

Thus, even if future, Kirby-like studies produce new evidence that abstinence-only programs "do not work," there would nonetheless remain the complex and consequential issue of how best to define "effectiveness."

About values more than science

This philosophical point leads to a fourth and final observation concerning the past, present, and even future scientific research on school-based sex-education programs.

The question of how best to define "effectiveness" is at bottom a question of value-laden guiding philosophies. And as such, it is a question that cannot exclusively or even primarily be settled by empirical investigation—although it certainly can and should be informed by such investigation.

The final arbiter will thus have to be the prevailing moral and philosophical convictions of the American public. Indeed, the issue of sex education so thoroughly and necessarily entails value-laden assumptions concerning human development, sexual identity and lifestyle, personal character, and rights and responsibilities that it is highly doubtful that researchers can conduct their investigations into the "effectiveness" of school-based sex-education programs free of such assumptions.

If they can't, this would by no means render their research worthless. It would suggest, however, that in many cases researchers—several of whom, including Kirby, publicly decried the recent federally mandated abstinence-only initiative for lacking sufficient empirical support—themselves may not be evaluating, and perhaps cannot evaluate, these programs in the roles of completely neutral, disinterested observers.

Quantifying the statistical regularities of teen pregnancy and STDs is one thing. But evaluating how best to educate teens about their sexual identity, development, and behavior is quite another—a necessarily and deeply value-laden thing.

Organizations to Contact

The editors have compiled the following list of organizations concerned with the issues debated in this book. The descriptions are derived from materials provided by the organizations. All have publications or information available for interested readers. The list was compiled on the date of publication of the present volume; the information provided here may change. Be aware that many organizations take several weeks or longer to respond to inquiries, so allow as much time as possible.

The Alan Guttmacher Institute
120 Wall St., New York, NY 10005
(212) 248-1111 • fax: (212) 248-1951
e-mail: info@agi-usa.org • website: http://www.agi-usa.org

The institute works to protect and expand the reproductive choices of all women and men. It strives to ensure that people have access to the information and services they need to exercise their rights and responsibilities concerning sexual activity, reproduction, and family planning. Among the institute's publications are the books *Teenage Pregnancy in Industrialized Countries* and *Today's Adolescents, Tomorrow's Parents: A Portrait of the Americas* and the report *Sex and America's Teenagers*.

Coalition for Positive Sexuality (CPS)
3712 N. Broadway, Suite 191, Chicago, IL 60613
(312) 604-1654
e-mail: cps@positive.org • website: http://www.positive.org/cps/

CPS is a grassroots volunteer group that joins local high school students with several national activist groups. Their purpose is to give teens vital information about sexuality and to facilitate dialogue in and out of the public schools on condom availability and sex education. CPS publishes the booklet *Just Say Yes!*, available in English and Spanish.

National Campaign to Prevent Teen Pregnancy
2100 M St. NW, Suite 300, Washington, DC 20037
(202) 261-5655
e-mail: campaign@teenpregnancy.org
website: http://www.teenpregnancy.org

The mission of the National Campaign is to reduce teenage pregnancy by supporting values and stimulating actions that are consistent with a pregnancy-free adolescence. The campaign's goal is to reduce the pregnancy rate among teenage girls by one-third by the year 2005. The campaign publishes pamphlets, brochures, and opinion polls such as: *No Easy Answers: Research Finding on Programs to Reduce Teen Pregnancy, Not Just for Girls: Involving Boys and Men in Teen Pregnancy Prevention,* and *Public Opinion Polls and Teen Pregnancy.*

National Organization on Adolescent Pregnancy, Parenting, and Prevention (NOAPPP)
1319 F St. NW, Suite 400, Washington, DC 20004
(202) 783-5770 • fax: (202) 783-5775
website: http://www.noappp.org

NOAPPP's mission is to provide leadership, education, training, information and advocacy resources, and support to practitioners in the field. Believing that the entire community is essential to successfully addressing adolescent pregnancy, NOAPPP provides a forum where divergent viewpoints can be expressed and valued and common ground can be cleared for action. NOAPPP does not represent any single political perspective, curriculum, program model, or policy approach. Its publications include *Kids Having Kids, Trying to Maximize the Odds: Using What We Know to Prevent Teen Pregnancy*, and the *NOAPPP Newsletter*.

Planned Parenthood Federation of America
810 Seventh Ave., New York, NY 10019
(212) 541-7800 • fax: (212) 245-1845
e-mail: communications@ppfa.org
website: http://www.plannedparenthood.org

Planned Parenthood believes that all individuals should have access to comprehensive sexuality education in order to make decisions about their own fertility. It provides contraception, abortion, and family planning services at clinics located throughout the United States. Among its extensive publications are the fact sheets *Helping Young People to Delay Sexual Intercourse, Pregnancy and Childbearing Among U.S. Teens*, and *Reducing Teenage Pregnancy*.

Sexuality Information and Education Council of the United States (SIECUS)
130 W. 42nd St., Suite 350, New York, NY 10036-7802
(212) 819-9770 • fax: (212) 819-9776
e-mail: siecus@siecus.org • website: http://www.siecus.org

SIECUS is a clearinghouse for information on sexuality, with a special interest in sex education. It publishes sex education curricula, the bimonthly newsletter *SIECUS Report*, and fact sheets on sex education issues. Its articles, bibliographies, and book reviews often address the role of sex education in reducing and preventing teen sexual activity.

Teen-Aid
723 E. Jackson Ave., Spokane, WA 99207
(509) 482-2868 • fax: (509) 482-7994
e-mail: teenaid@teen-aid.org • website: http://www.teen-aid.org

Teen-Aid is a not-for-profit corporation whose purpose is to promote premarital abstinence in schools through parent-teen communication. It teaches the skills needed to reinforce character and family values. The main curricula developed by Teen-Aid cover general and reproductive health, parenting skills, birth control information, refusal skills, sexually transmitted disease information, sexual harassment, abuse, and date rape. Teen-Aid has online publications that can be accessed through their website.

Bibliography

Books

Eleanor Ayer	*It's Okay to Say No: Choosing Sexual Abstinence.* New York: Rosen, 1997.
Brent A. Barlow	*Worth Waiting for: Sexual Abstinence Before Marriage.* Salt Lake City, UT: Deseret, 1995.
Michael J. Basso	*The Underground Guide to Teenage Sexuality: An Essential Handbook for Today's Teen and Parents.* Minneapolis, MN: Fairview Press, 1997.
Ruth Bell	*Changing Bodies, Changing Lives: A Book for Teens on Sex and Relationships.* New York: Times Books, 1998.
Jon Knowles and Marcia Ringel	*All About Birth Control: A Personal Guide.* New York: Three Rivers Press, 1998.
Kristin Luker	*Dubious Conceptions: The Politics of Teenage Pregnancy.* Cambridge, MA: Harvard University Press, 1996.
Patricia F. Miller	*Sex Is Not a Four-Letter Word!: Talking Sex with Your Children Made Easier.* New York: Crossroad, 1995.
Barbaro Moe	*Everything You Need to Know About Sexual Abstinence.* New York: Rosen, 1998.
Ronald Filiberti Moglia and Jon Knowles, eds.	*All About Sex: A Family Resource on Sex and Sexuality.* New York: Crown, 1997.
Kristin M. Napier	*The Power of Abstinence.* New York: Avon, 1996.
Jeffery S. Nevid and Fern Gotfried	*Choices: Sex in the Age of STDs.* Needham Heights, MA: Allyn & Bacon, 1995.
Richard A. Panzer	*Condom Nation: Blind Faith, Bad Science.* Westwood, NJ: Center for Educational Media, 1997.
Cindy Patton	*Fatal Advice: How Safe-Sex Education Went Wrong.* Durham, NC: Duke University Press, 1996.
Ira L. Reiss and Harriet M. Reiss	*Solving America's Sexual Crises.* Amherst, NY: Prometheus, 1997.

Periodicals

Mary Abowd	"What Are Your Kids Learning About Sex?" *U.S. Catholic,* April 1996.
Eric Alterman	"Neutering America," *Nation,* February 19, 1996.
Alison Bell	"Sex Education Now . . . or Never?" *Sassy,* September 1996.

Linda A. Berne and Barbara K. Huberman — "Sexuality Education: Sorting Fact from Fiction," *Phi Delta Kappan*, November 1995.

Tom Bethell — "Smoking and Sex," *National Review*, May 19, 1997.

Francesca Delbanco — "No Sex Ed," *Seventeen*, October 1997.

M. Joycelyn Elders — "Respect Your Elders! Abstinence Is Hazardous to Our Nation's Youth," *POZ*, December 1997. Available from 349 W. Twelfth St., New York, NY 10014-1721.

David Friedman — "Look Who's Teaching Sex," *Good Housekeeping*, November 1996.

Katherine Griffin — "Sex Education That Works," *Health*, May/June 1995.

William Norman Grigg — "They Want Your Children," *New American*, June 8, 1998. Available from 770 Westhill Blvd., Appleton, WI 54914.

William Jasper — "Joycelyn Elders' Last Words," *New American*, January 23, 1995.

Peter LaBarbera — "NEA Pushes Homosexual Agenda," *Christian American*, May 1995. Available from Christian Coalition, 1801-L Sara Dr., Chesapeake, VA 23320.

Joe Loconte — "A City's Assault on Teen Pregnancy," *Policy Review*, November/December 1996.

Mindszenty Report — "Sex Education: You Can Say No," October 1996.

J. Jennings Moss — "Classroom Warfare," *Advocate*, March 4, 1997.

Richard Nadler — "Abstaining from Sex Education," *National Review*, September 15, 1997.

Lynn Rosellini — "Joycelyn Elders Is Master of Her Domain," *U.S. News & World Report*, November 3, 1997.

Jeannie I. Rosoff — "Helping Teenagers Avoid Negative Consequences of Sexual Activity," *USA Today*, May 1996.

Annys Shin — "Abstinence-Only Programs Get the Big Bucks," *Ms.*, January/February 1998.

SIECUS Report — Issue Theme: Sex Education, August/September 1997. Available from 130 W. 142nd St., Suite 350, New York, NY 10036-7802.

Alan Singer — "Preaching Ain't Teaching," *Rethinking Schools*, Winter 1996–1997.

Ron Stodghill II — "Where'd You Learn That?" *Time*, June 15, 1998.

Jeff Stryker — "Abstinence or Else!" *Nation*, June 16, 1997.

Meredith Tax — "My Censorship—and Ours," *Nation*, March 20, 1995.

Barbara Dafoe Whitehead — "The Failure of Sex Education," *Atlantic Monthly*, October 1994.

Paula Wilson — "Rise and Fall of the Surgeon General," *USA Today*, May 1997.

Index